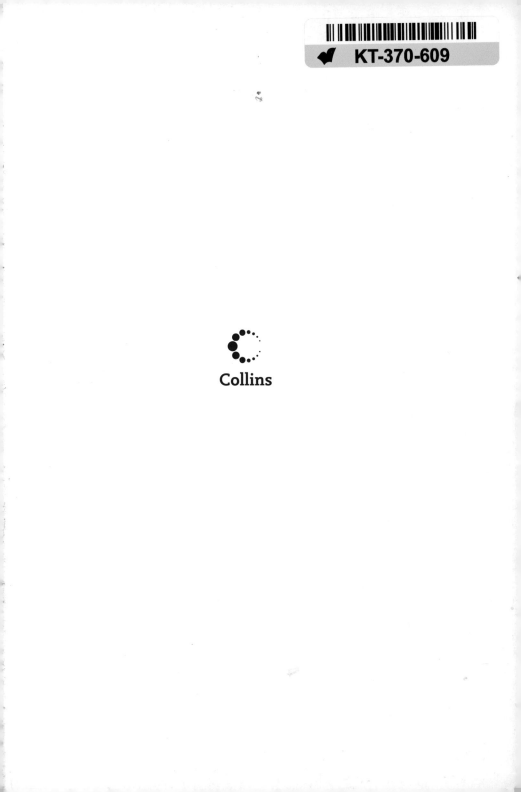

Collins

need to know?

GI+GL
Diet

Collins

First published in 2006 by Collins
an imprint of
HarperCollins Publishers
77-85 Fulham Palace Road
London W6 8JB

www.collins.co.uk

A catalogue record for this book is available from
the British Library

Project management: Grapevine Publishing Services
Text: Kate Santon
Designer: Judith Ash
Cover photographs: © Corbis

ISBN 0-00-7219911

Printed and bound by Printing Express Ltd,
Hong Kong

Contents

Introduction

There have been many attempts to develop the perfect diet, one that would make losing weight both easy and relatively painless. Can GI+GL tick all the boxes?

Why choose GI+GL?

Some diets have been restrictive, requiring dieters to eat quantities of one particular food – like cabbage soup, grapefruit or pineapple. Others, a bit more complicated, have essentially recommended cutting out a whole group of foods, as the original Atkins diet did with carbohydrates. Some have suggested that only ever eating certain types of food in particular combinations might do the trick. Or you might need to consider physical factors like your blood type in detail...

It often seems as though new diets appear every day. Many of them stress the disadvantages of all the previous diet plans, and spend a lot of time doing this. Sometimes they seem to exist to push just one, very strongly held, dieting theory which may be decidedly strange but is being publicised by a celebrity fan. And these diets seem to be getting much more complicated and much more limiting.

Recent versions of the Atkins diet have addressed this tendency and become less restrictive, allowing some non-starchy carbohydrates. However, there's still an initial phase when you cut out carbs so completely that your body burns fat for the fuel it needs, a state known as ketosis. Many doctors have expressed their fears about this, feeling that essential foods, like fruit or whole grains, should not be restricted in this way. There were even some deaths blamed on the diet, after dieters suffered severe metabolic imbalances, and consequently

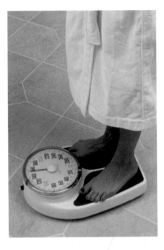

high-protein diets received a lot of negative publicity.

Make sure your scales are calibrated, for a more accurate reading.

Many Atkins dieters were losing weight, often very quickly and dramatically. They did tend to have bad breath from the ketosis, constipation and a general feeling of being unwell; some reported severe headaches and dizzy fits. But when they stopped the diet, whether they'd achieved their target weight or not, the kilos piled back on. Latest news is that Atkins Nutritional has filed for bankruptcy in the US.

That's the way it so often is. Most diets do work – in the beginning, and if you stick to them religiously. But most are boring, most leave you feeling ravenous and then guilty when you give in to temptation. In addition they may make you feel ill, faint and unfit. Failure is almost inevitable; you'd need a will of iron to hang on in these circumstances. And when you do stop, any weight you've lost just zaps back on. There's a reason for this. If a diet involves restricting the amount of food you eat, and they almost all do, then your body adjusts. It gets used to having less food and your resting metabolic rate drops: your body needs less energy, in the form of food, just to keep its basic processes – like breathing or blood circulation – going. When you go back to eating normally, you put weight on easily because your body has got used to requiring less food, and stores it in the form of fat instead of using it as necessary fuel.

Everyone who is deliberately trying to lose weight, for whatever reason, knows how very difficult it is. Sticking to a restrictive, severe or limiting plan makes it very likely that even the most determined dieters will be tempted to drift away from

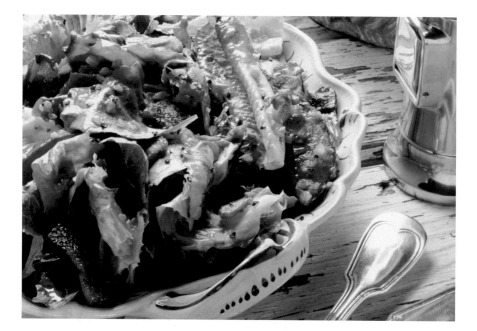

what they are supposed to be eating. Very few diets stress the importance of enjoying the food you eat. Maybe what most dieters need is something that isn't a 'diet'. This is where the GI diet and its close relative the GL diet come in. They work because they're enjoyable. They provide a way of eating for life, one which is healthy and which will help you lose weight, if you are careful. People who follow the rules lose weight slowly and steadily – and keep it off, too.

What's more, doctors and nutritionists approve of the GI diet. It's not extreme and it doesn't forbid important categories of food like carbohydrates or fat (we all need some fat in our diet for our bodies to function). The World Health Organisation has suggested that it is good for your health. Some GI-based diets have been developed by medics, particularly cardiologists and those working with diabetics, or by scientists and fully qualified nutritionists. This might make it sound as though a GI diet was going to be complicated to follow, requiring a lot of maths,

It's not all lettuce leaves and hunger pangs on the GI+GL diet,

weighing scales and a calculator, but this is another great benefit of the GI diet – it's easy. You don't need to do lots of careful weighing; you don't need to tot up calories, grams of fat, calculate 'points' or anything like that. You do have to understand a bit of basic nutrition, and you need to bear that in mind as you cook and eat. You also have to keep an eye on portion sizes, but in a simple, straightforward way.

The food tastes great, it doesn't leave you desperate for something to eat between meals, you don't have to weigh food all the time or count up the calories it contains. A GI+GL diet isn't tiresomely restrictive and it can easily be adapted to include many favourite dishes, or to suit different tastes and food preferences. In addition, eating like this can help your health. In fact, many doctors and nutritionists have described the GI diet as a simple return to healthy eating, to eating in the way we did before we all came to rely on convenience and processed foods and ingredients. It reduces the risk of developing diabetes or having a heart attack, improves your overall health and increases your energy levels. It soon becomes second nature because it's actually enjoyable. Hopefully you'll barely notice that you're dieting!

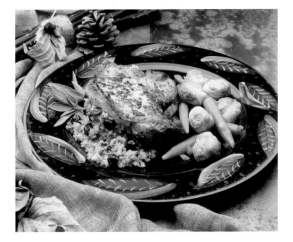

GI/GL meals contain a little starchy carb, some protein and lots of vegetables.

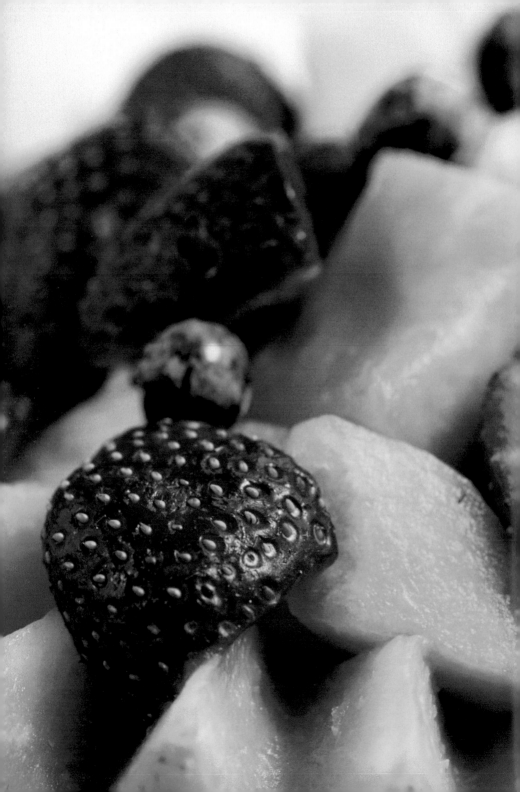

1 How does it work?

Now for the science. It's not tricky to follow. You'll probably find that you recognise the effects different types of food have on your blood sugar and energy levels, because you've been noticing it yourself for years. Ever felt you needed an afternoon nap after a lunch of pizza and garlic bread? Does that 4pm Danish pastry really get you through the rest of the working day? Help yourself by regulating your blood sugar and gaining energy at the same time.

How does it work?

Food has an effect on the way your body works. Nobody doubts that. The key to the success of the GI diet is that it uses your body's natural responses to help you lose weight.

Pizzas are high GI, causing blood sugar to peak then plummet.

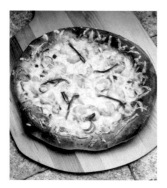

What happens when we eat?

When you eat starchy carbohydrates like bread, cereals, pasta or potatoes, your body digests the starch they contain. This becomes glucose – sugar – and is then used by the body as a source of energy.

In digestion, all foods are broken down into molecules which can be absorbed by the body. This process happens in the digestive tract, where enzymes are secreted which break down the food into its component parts. Most digestion happens in the small intestine, but some 'simple' foods are digested in the stomach itself. Glucose is one, and as a result it enters the bloodstream rapidly. The level of glucose in the blood then shoots up. (You can imagine how fast this happens, because alcohol is also digested in the stomach and everyone knows how quickly you can get drunk, especially on an empty stomach.)

Why does blood sugar matter?

The rapid rise in the level of glucose in the blood can be followed by an equally rapid fall, which sends a signal to your body telling it to boost the glucose level again. This is why you often feel hungry soon after eating something that causes a rapid rise in glucose. So grabbing a chocolate bar when you're hungry might make you feel better for a while, but

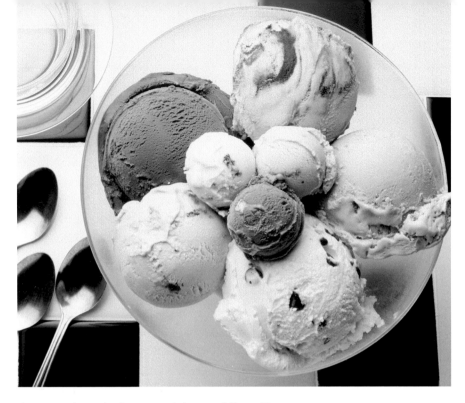

Most icecreams are high
GI, high GL and high
calorie.

the energy boost is short term. It is soon followed by a drop in blood sugar levels, making you feel hungrier than ever.

This is where insulin becomes part of the picture. Insulin is a hormone generated in the pancreas which helps glucose enter the cells of your body where it can be used as energy. Most people have heard of insulin; it is the substance lacking in people with type 1 diabetes, which they need to inject every day if they are to survive. But many other people have the opposite problem with insulin – they have too much circulating in their blood. In fact, it is possible to develop a resistance to insulin, known as insulin resistance syndrome, syndrome X or metabolic syndrome. If you are resistant to insulin, then your body just produces more and more, trying to provoke the correct response.

weblinks: www.diabetes.org.uk

This is important because if you have high insulin levels you are likely to get fatter, whatever steps you take to reduce your weight. The higher the level of insulin, the more carbohydrate your body uses up – and the lower the amount of fat it uses. This is because insulin doesn't just make it possible for glucose to enter the cells of the body; it also inhibits the release of stored fat. So stabilising insulin levels is essential, and to do that you have to stabilise your blood sugar levels. It is crucial to keep your blood sugar levels on an even keel if you want to lose weight.

What diabetics know
Diabetics have known about the importance of insulin for a long time, but certain recent changes in the way the condition is managed can be useful for those who want to lose weight. There are two types of diabetes. People with type 1 diabetes don't produce insulin at all; their injections keep them alive. Type 2 diabetes is more common and generally develops later in life, though there are now some cases occurring in children. Worryingly, one of the risk factors for developing it is simply being overweight or obese.

People with type 2 diabetes fail to produce enough insulin for their bodies, but they can usually manage to control their condition by modifying what they eat, or by the combination of healthy eating and medication. There's no such thing as 'mild' diabetes – the consequences of both types can be severe – and the main consideration of all diabetics is to avoid highs and lows in their blood sugar levels.

Diabetics used to be recommended to eat a diet rich in starchy carbs. However, recent studies have shown that these carbs release their sugar into the bloodstream too quickly, resulting in surges in blood sugar levels known as 'spikes'. These surges can lead to collapse, so it was important for doctors to understand more. Scientists and researchers began to realise that not all carbs produced blood sugar rushes because some were broken down more slowly, and they started systematic testing. Controlled scientific trials produced an interesting result: far better for diabetics were those foods that were much less disruptive to the level of blood sugar. Eating food that was more slowly absorbed by the digestive system could smooth out blood sugar levels over the whole day.

The glycaemic index, or GI, developed out of all the testing that was being carried out in several centres worldwide in the 1980s and 90s. Then the concept of the GL – glycaemic load – was also developed, to modify some of the shortcomings of the GI, and has been gaining credibility in the diabetic community when used together with the GI. Trials with diabetics have now specifically shown that a diet with a low GI improves blood sugar control, and scientists have stressed that high GI foods are best avoided. Other researchers were also developing their ideas, and the whole idea of using the GI more generally began to snowball.

Could you pick the foods from the picture below that would give you a blood sugar spike?

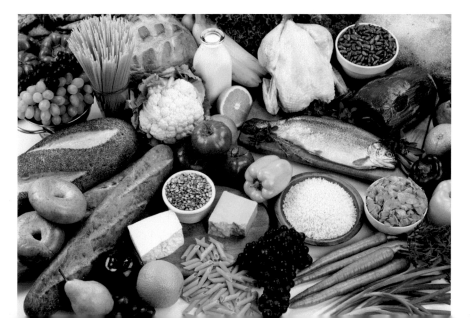

The glycaemic index

The GI is a numerical system that indicates how quickly a specific food will trigger a rise in the level of blood sugar. Researchers began to give relative scores to the different types of carbs they were testing, according to how quickly they were converted into blood sugar, and these scores became known as the glycaemic index. Foods with a low GI (under 55) break down slowly, giving a slow rise in blood sugar and insulin levels; high GI foods – like white bread – break down much more quickly, sending both blood sugar and insulin levels surging upwards.

How is the GI value decided?

Carbs are rated by testing precisely measured portions of food on ten or more healthy people first thing in the morning, before they have eaten anything else. The food they are given is usually a portion which contains 50g of carbs, so that the relative rises in blood sugar levels caused by different foods can be assessed against each other. Over the next two hours the human guinea pigs have their blood sugar levels monitored at specific intervals. The results are then used to plot a curve on a graph for the food being tested. This curve is assessed against a reference food – glucose in most testing centres, but sometimes white bread – which is given a value of 100.

must know

Shopping
Go food shopping after a meal – looking for things to eat on an empty stomach is fatal for anyone's diet!

High, medium or low?

Every food has a specific numerical GI value, but for practical, everyday purposes it is much more convenient to divide foods into high, medium and low GI.

High GI foods have a value of 70 or more. They include white bread, chips, easy-cook rice, cakes, biscuits, chocolate and a lot of processed foods. Cornflakes, for example, have a GI of 84, while a basic muesli is just 56.

The glucose process

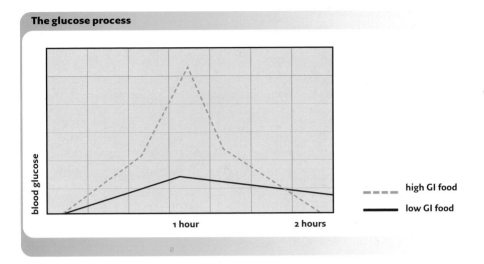

blood glucose

1 hour   2 hours

- - - - high GI food
———— low GI food

Medium GI foods have a GI value of between 56 and 69. They include things like rye crispbreads, figs and bananas, and bran-based or multigrain cereals.

Low GI foods are the most important for anyone trying to control their weight and are the ones you are supposed to favour on the GI diet. They include many vegetables and a lot of fruit – cherries have a GI of 22 – beans, pulses... and lots more.

These categories are often given a traffic-light coding: red for 'high and hardly ever', amber or yellow for 'medium and maybe', and green for 'low and go'.

Quick and easy clues

There are a couple of basic guidelines which you can use to distinguish between 'good' and 'bad' carbs, as some people call them – though, as many nutritionists have pointed out, 'good' and 'bad' aren't really helpful words to use. It's the proportion of them in the diet that's the problem, not the carb itself.

Firstly, taste is a good guide. The sweeter something is, the more quickly you'll get a blood sugar surge when you eat it. Sugars – simple

must know

Pulses and beans
These have a reputation for causing flatulence. If you do start suffering from excessive wind, don't stop eating them; your body will adapt quite quickly.

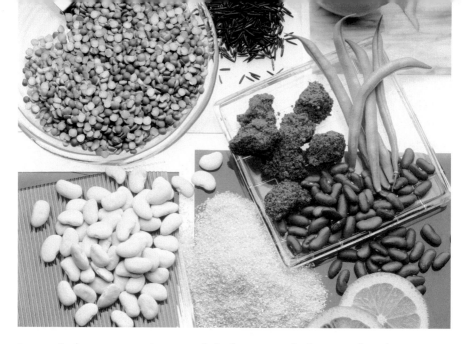

Beans and pulses tend to have low GI and GL values.

carbohydrates – are the fastest carbs to be converted to blood glucose.

Then there's fibre. Carbs like whole grains, beans, seeds, pulses and some vegetables are much, much slower to be broken down, and one of the things that slows them down is the amount of fibre they contain. Refined, processed foods, like white flour, cakes, biscuits or rice which is treated to make it easier to cook, are also relatively quick to be converted as the processes they are subjected to in manufacture remove a lot of their fibre. Complex carbs like whole grains need to be broken down and therefore take some time to be absorbed into the bloodstream. The result is a slower rise in blood sugar levels.

The GI is especially valuable because it encourages healthy eating, and that doesn't just mean a loss in weight. Low GI diets have also been shown to lower the risk of developing heart disease and type 2 diabetes. One word of warning, though –

food only has a GI if it contains carbohydrate. If you are hoping to lose weight, you do have to bear in mind that some no-GI foods are very high in calories. Butter has no GI value, but that doesn't mean that you can eat a lot of it without gaining weight.

So far, so straightforward. But nothing is quite that simple.

Limitations of the GI

The GI of a meal is affected by the way food is cooked, and by any other ingredients used, especially the amount of fat and protein eaten at the same time. These all influence the overall GI of the meal, and can reduce the effect of one of the items having a high GI value. It is possible to go into a lot of detail about this, but you really don't need to. It's plain common sense – yes, adding lots of butter to your bread may reduce the overall GI of your snack, as would toasting the bread first, but it still won't do a lot for reducing your waistline.

The biggest problem is that, in isolation, GI values fail to take any account of actual portion sizes. This is a consequence of the way they were established in the first place. To give a valid comparison, which is very important, the human guinea pigs used in testing were given portions of each food that contained 50g of carbohydrate. This failed to take into account realistic portion sizes. To get 50g of carbs in sugar you wouldn't need a very big portion (just 10 teaspoons), but to get the same carb content with a green, leafy vegetable you'd need much more. Very much more. In fact, eating a test portion of broccoli – one which contained 50g of

must know

Breakfast
Breakfast is the first and most important meal of the day, as during the night your blood sugar levels will have dropped. It's important to refuel in the morning or you risk hunger pangs, shakiness and snacking before lunchtime.

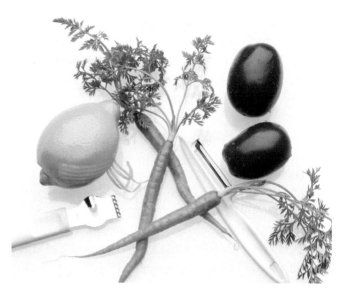

Only peel fruits and vegetables if the peel is inedible. The extra fibre in peel lowers the overall GI value.

carbohydrate – isn't something you'd be likely to do in everyday life at all: it would be about 5 kilos.

So, as the GI in isolation can sometimes be misleading, another measurement has been developed – the GL.

The glycaemic load

There are some very clear examples of why it's not a good idea to rely on the GI alone. For instance, brazil nuts and broccoli are both low GI foods, but 50g of brazil nuts contains 157 calories, and the same quantity of broccoli has 10.5. Or take carrots. They have a similar GI to some jams, but you would have to eat dozens of carrots for them to have a significant effect on your blood sugar levels, while even a spoonful of jam would give you a blood sugar spike almost immediately. Some medium GI foods which are particularly carbohydrate dense, like basmati rice or some wheat-flour pastas, can increase blood sugar levels substantially. The body still has to deal with a large 'load' of carbs. Examples such as these have led to much discussion about the value of using the GI by itself.

The glycaemic load goes a step further by considering the amount of carbohydrate an individual is actually likely to eat. A GL value is worked out by multiplying the GI value of the food concerned by the number of grams of carbohydrate it contains in a usual serving, and then dividing the total by a hundred.

GI value x grams of carb per serving ÷ 100 = GL value

GL values are much lower numerically than those of the GI. A food with a high GL has a value of 20 or more, while one with a medium GL falls in the 11-19 range, and a low GL food would have a value of 10 or less. As with the GI, for practical reasons these are often just called high, medium or low, and given the same red, yellow and green traffic-light coding.

Differences between GI and GL values

There are some discrepancies that arise when portion size is taken into consideration. Some medium GI foods that are particularly carbohydrate dense can substantially increase blood sugar and insulin levels if you eat enough, and 'enough' doesn't have to be that much – two cups of cooked, wheat-based pasta has a very high GL.

Broccoli is an excellent source of vitamin C and folic acid.

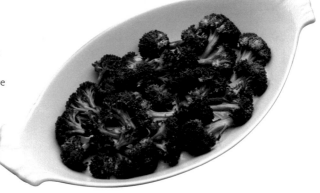

must know

The diet habit
Habits can be good for you. It takes about three weeks for a repetitive action to become a habit, so do your best not to give up dieting too early.

must know

Fruit juice
Fruit juices can be high in calories, and also have a high GI because they don't contain as much fibre as the whole fruit. Try to avoid them, or drink them heavily diluted.

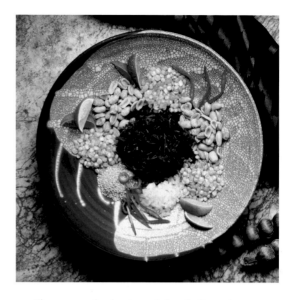

Nuts and seeds are an important source of essential fatty acids as well as a low GI/GL snack.

The reverse is also true. A few fruits and vegetables have a high GI but once quantity is considered, using their GL instead, the picture is rather different:

	GI value	GL value
Cantaloupe melon	65	4
Watermelon	72	4
Pumpkin	75	3
Broad beans, cooked	80	9

There are other discrepancies. Carrots have a medium GI but a low GL, for example.

GI or GL? Or both?
Some nutritionists think that the GL is an improvement on the GI because it considers quantity as well as quality. However, both values have been found to work together in large-scale studies at Harvard University. The risk of disease was

predicted by the overall GI of the diet as well as its glycaemic load, and the Harvard Group therefore recommended that people should focus on wholegrains and minimise their intake of potatoes and rice. The use of the GL reinforced the relationship between a GI diet and good health.

Most nutritionists and dietitians stress that it is important not to use the GL by itself. If you did, you could very easily end up eating large amounts of protein and significant quantities of fat, but without enough carbohydrate for a balanced diet. Choose carbs that are slowly digested (with a low GI) over those that are broken down more quickly, even if they have an identical GL. The overall aim should be to improve the quality of the carbs eaten.

The GL has its uses, though. You can use it to compare similar foods – different kinds of bread, perhaps – and discover which is the best for your diet. If you were trying to decide between cantaloupe melon and chocolate, then the GL would be a good guide (mind you, so would common sense!).

The GL really comes into its own in identifying the exceptions to the GI, the places where the quantity you'd have to eat to match the test quantities would be huge, like watermelon, pumpkin, cantaloupe and broad beans. Bear both in mind when you are dieting, but be sensible – that's the best advice from dietitians andnutritionists.

More basic GI+GL diet rules
Once you understand more about how your digestion works, you can use it to your advantage. Here are some basic guidelines to bear in mind.

must know

Keep your balance
Overall balance is the key to healthy eating, and to losing weight healthily, too. Fad diets don't help, and may cause more problems. You need a whole variety of nutrients to stay well.

▶ It's important that rises and falls in blood sugar are as gentle as possible if you want to lose weight, so the longer the process of digestion takes, the better. Fibre slows the absorption of sugars during digestion. Wholegrain products, which keep their fibre content, are lower in GI than their refined, white product equivalents, which have had most of their fibre removed. When your body has to digest carbs with a tougher coat, like wholegrains, then they take longer to cause rises in blood sugar. If something is peeled, ground, mashed, puréed or processed before being eaten then it is much more easily broken down into glucose. It's easy to understand this if you imagine how quickly your body would digest a cream of vegetable soup, then think about how long it would take to digest all the raw vegetables it contains. The same principle applies to other things, too. An entire fruit or vegetable is always lower in GI than its juice, for example.

Orange juice has a higher GI value (50) than the fruit itself (which is 42).

- Some starches are more easily broken down in the digestive system than others. This is why some similar types of food have different GI values: basmati rice is harder to digest than white rice, so it has a lower GI. If the starch granules in a food have swollen and burst, then that food will be digested very quickly; if they are still in their 'raw' state then digestion will be slower.
- Cooking can affect GI values. The longer a vegetable is boiled, the less fibre it retains. Cooking things quickly and eating them while they still have some crunch means more work for your digestive system.
- Fats and proteins slow the digestion of carbohydrate, and reduce the effects of high-GI food on blood sugar.
So if you have a boiled egg with your wholemeal toast, your breakfast will have a lower GI than if you'd chosen jam, marmalade or fruit spread. This is also why crisps have a lower GI than baked potatoes – but eating lots of crisps is still not a good idea!
- Consider the meal as a whole. If you combine a high GI food with a low one, then the overall effect will be medium GI. This can be useful to remember when you are eating out or when you have little choice about what you are offered; you can moderate the effects of something which has a high GI by being selective.
- Acids also reduce GI value, so if you sprinkle lemon juice over your meal, or a little vinegar, you will reduce the overall GI. In practice this can mean something like having a vinaigrette – home-made not bottled, for preference, as bottled ones often contain sugar – with your salad if you are also eating bread.
- Finally, remember that the GI and the GL only measure the effect of carbs. They don't measure calories, fats, proteins – so portion control is critical. We'll get on to that!

want to know more?

- To find out if you are diabetic or suffer from pre-diabetes or syndrome X, ask your doctor to refer you for a simple blood test.
- For advice on diabetes, contact Diabetes UK on 0845 1202960 or visit their website www.diabetes.org.uk
- To find GI ratings for common foods in the UK, see *Collins Gem GI guide*. Many basics are listed in chapter 9 of this book.
- More GI values for basic foods can be found at www.glycaemicindex.com
- Jennie Brand-Miller's book *The Complete Guide to GI Values* and her website www.glycemicindex.com provide GI ratings, but focus on foods for sale in Australia rather than the UK.
- See page 190 for a range of GI and GL diets available in bookshops.

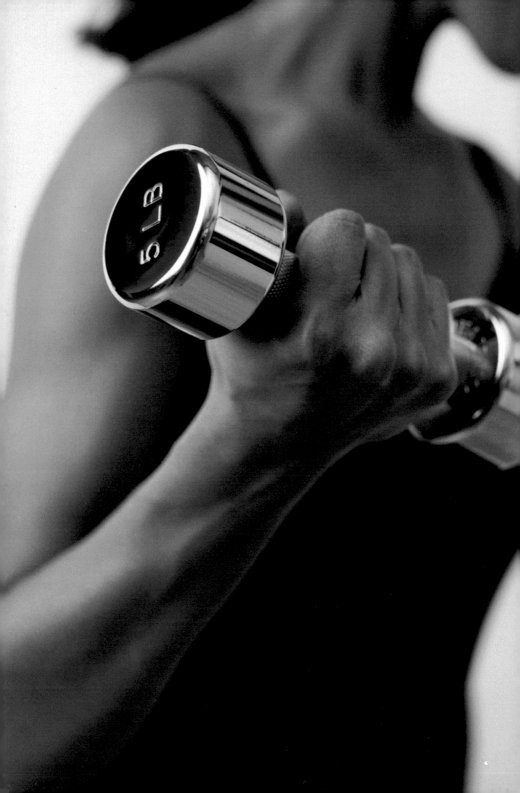

2 Losing weight

How much weight will you lose on a GI+GL diet, and how quickly will you lose it? These are the questions every dieter wants to ask, but the answers are individual, depending on your body shape, the amount of body fat you have, your metabolism and how active you are, among other factors. In this chapter, you'll discover what would be a sensible and realistic rate of weight loss for you.

Losing weight

The first thing to do before starting any diet is to work out how much you really need to lose. Everyone is different, so there are no cut-and-dried rules for how much you should weigh.

must know

Aim small
Even minor losses in weight can result in better health, and losing little by little, over time, means you're more likely to keep the weight off.

How much should you lose?

Women have a tendency to think they need to lose more than they really do, and the media frequently focus on a stick-thin ideal which would be actively unhealthy for the majority of people. Men tend to be more accurate about their weight, but don't always believe they need to do anything about it: 'dieting's for wimps.' They're wrong...

The first thing to do before starting any diet is to work out how much you really need to lose. Everyone is different, so there are no across-the-board rules about how much you should weigh. Time to try and be objective. Consider your overall build. If you have a naturally large frame – big shoulders, broad hips – then you'll never turn yourself into someone with a tiny frame, no matter how little you eat. If you're a woman with a naturally curvy figure, you'll never transform yourself into a straight-up-straight-down stick insect. Some of our predispositions are genetic; we'll never, ever alter them. And one of the things we all have a genetic predispostion for is a particular weight range.

If you consume more energy in the form of food than you use up in the form of exercise, then you'll start to gain weight above that range, because excess energy is stored as fat. If you consume less energy than you use, then you'll drop below that range, and that's not necessarily a good thing. If you diet down to a weight lower than your natural range, you'll find it almost impossible to maintain.

Standard body weight for height and frame size

Men

Height m (ft)	Small Frame kg (lbs)	Medium Frame kg (lbs)	Large Frame kg (lbs)
1.60 (5'3")	51–61 (113–134)	54–64 (119–140)	58–68 (127–150)
1 63 (5'4")	53–61 (116–135)	55–65 (122–142)	59–70 (131–154)
1.65 (5'5")	54–62 (119–137)	57–66 (125–146)	60–72 (133–159)
1.68 (5'6")	56–64 (123–140)	59–68 (129–149)	62–74 (137–163)
1.70 (5'7")	58–65 (127–143)	60–69 (133–152)	64–76 (142–167)
1.73 (5'8")	60–66 (131–145)	62–71 (137–155)	66–78 (146–171)
1.75 (5'9")	61–68 (135–149)	64–72 (141–158)	68–80 (150–175)
1.78 (5'10")	63–69 (139–152)	66–73 (145–161)	70–81 (154–179)
1.80 (5'11")	65–70 (143–155)	68–75 (149–165)	72–83 (159–183)
1.83 (6")	67–72 (147–159)	70–77 (153–169)	74–85 (163–187)
1.85 (6'1")	69–75 (151–165)	71–80 (157–175)	76–86 (167–189)
1.88 (6'2')	70–76 (155–168)	73–81 (161–179)	78–89 (171–197)
1.90 (6'3")	72–79 (157–173)	75–84 (166–185)	80–92 (176–202)

Women

Height m (ft)	Small Frame kg (lbs)	Medium Frame kg (lbs)	Large Frame kg (lbs)
1.50 (4'11")	42–51 (93–112)	44–55 (98–121)	48–57 (106–125)
1.52 (5')	44–52 (96–115)	46–57 (101–124)	49–58 (109–128)
1.55 (5'1")	45–54 (99–118)	47–58 (104–127)	51–59 (112–131)
1.57 (5'2")	46–55 (102–121)	49–60 (107–132)	52–61 (115–135)
1.60 (5'3")	48–56 (105–124)	50–62 (110–135)	54–63 (118–138)
1.63 (5'4")	49–58 (108–127)	51–63 (113–138)	55–65 (122–142)
1.65 (5'5")	50–59 (111–130)	53–64 (117–141)	57–66 (126–145)
1.68 (5'6")	52–60 (115–133)	55–66 (121–144)	59–67 (130–148)
1.70 (5'7")	54–62 (119–136)	57–67 (125–147)	61–69 (134–151)
1.73 (5'8")	56–63 (123–139)	58–68 (128–150)	62–71 (137–155)
1.75 (5'9")	58–64 (127–142)	60–69 (133–153)	64–73 (141–159)
1.78 (5'10")	59–66 (131–145)	62–71 (137–156)	66–75 (146–165)
1.80 (5'11")	61–68 (135–148)	64–72 (141–159)	68–77 (150–170)
1.83 (6')	63–69 (138–151)	65–74 (143–163)	69–79 (153–173)

Ways of assessing weight

The most traditional way of seeing how much weight you need to lose is to consult a height and weight chart, like the one on page 29. These show the relationship between how tall you are and how much you weigh to suggest an 'ideal' weight.

Before using it, you need to decide whether you have a small, medium or large frame. One very rough way of checking is to circle the thumb and middle finger of one hand round the opposite wrist. If they overlap, you are likely to have a small frame; if they just touch, you have a medium frame, and if they don't meet, you could be large-framed.

Height and weight charts are a good starting point, but they don't really provide enough information. For one thing, they are only approximations, reflecting a very broad cultural average, and because of that there are many things which can distort their results. Muscle, for example, weighs more than fat, so somebody who exercises regularly might well appear to be overweight on a height/weight chart.

Body mass index

Nowadays doctors are more likely to use the body mass index (BMI) to judge weight. This is a way of assessing how much body fat someone is carrying, though there's still the same problem with those who have a lot of lean muscle mass.

You can work out your BMI by dividing your weight in kilograms by the square of your height in metres (it's not as complicated as it sounds, and there are some quick calculators and charts online which do the sums for you – see below right).

2.65

weight ÷ (height x height) = BMI

For example, if you were 1.65 m tall (5 ft 5 inches) and weighed 76 kg (12 stones), it would work out like this:

$$1.65 \times 1.65 = 2.72$$
$$76 \div 2.72 = 27.94$$

BMI figures are grouped into categories, so when you have worked yours out, check to see where you fit on this scale:

less than 15	**emaciated**
15–19	**underweight**
19–25	**average**
25–30	**overweight**
30–40	**obese**
over 40	**severely obese**

These BMI 'cutoffs' apply to healthy adults, not to pregnant women, those with certain medical conditions, the elderly or people under 18. Special charts have been developed for children and adolescents which take into account their age, level of growth and gender; if you are worried about a young person, then consult your doctor.

Additionally, BMI charts may not be appropriate for athletes, because of muscle weight distorting the figures. They are different for some ethnic groups – the World Health Organisation has, for instance, estimated that a BMI of 27.5 would carry the same health risk for an Asian as a BMI of 30 would for someone with a white Caucasian background. But the BMI does provide broad general guidelines which

must know

Sports drinks
Don't go anywhere near 'sports' drinks when you exercise; they are everything a GI dieter should avoid. They are specifically created to give instant energy – an immediate spike in blood-sugar levels – and the main ingredient is glucose.

weblinks: ww.eatwell.gov.uk/healthydiet/healthyweight/bmicalculator

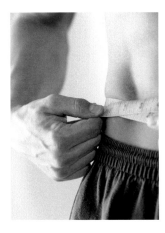

Waist circumference can be an indicator of health risks you face.

are useful, and you should certainly ask your doctor's advice if your BMI falls into the emaciated or obese range, as you could be endangering your health.

How big is your waist?

It's a serious question – the health problems associated with being overweight or obese aren't just a matter of excess fat, but of where that fat actually is. People with excess fat around their waists – who are often described as apple-shaped – are more at risk than those who are pear-shaped (fatter around their hips and thighs).

Abdominal fat isn't just a weight problem; in recent studies it's been shown to behave almost like another organ of the body, releasing fatty acids and harmful proteins which can increase the risk of heart disease, strokes, type 2 diabetes, and even cancer (in fact, obesity is second only to smoking as a cause of cancer). So the way your fat is distributed influences your health, and this is why doctors also consider waist-to-hip ratios and waist measurements.

To find your waist-to-hip ratio, divide your waist measurement by your hip measurement. If you're a man, and you get a figure above 1.0, then you are in the 'at risk' category, and if you're female you fall into that group if your number is above 0.85.

There are two levels of risk applied to waist measurements (and don't breathe in dramatically while measuring yourself!). If you're a woman, you're at risk of endangering your health if your waist is 80cm (32 in) or more, and at serious risk if it's more than 88cm (35 in). If you are a man, then your lower risk figure is 94cm (37 in), and you are putting your health at serious risk if it is 102cm (40 in) or over. The risk of heart disease is particularly marked.

must know

Catch the exercise habit
Exercising can feel as though you are fighting against instinct, but it can become a habit if you stick to it three times a week for at least three weeks.

Your ideal weight

The right weight for you is one at which you feel comfortable, energetic and, above all, healthy. Once you've got a BMI of between 19 and 25, you're at a healthy weight. If you are overweight, use the BMI to give you a rough target. How much weight would you need to lose to get into the average BMI range?

Time for a bit of maths again. Multiply the BMI you want to reach by the square of your height in metres, which you used to establish your current BMI: that will give you the weight you'd need to be. Let's take the example of someone whose BMI worked out at 27.94, described earlier. There the height squared was 2.72 and this person wants to reach a BMI of 25, so:

2.72 x 25 (desired BMI) = 68 (the weight in kilos which matches it)

Finally, subtract what you want to weigh from what you actually do weigh to find out how much you need to lose to reach a healthier BMI – for this person the target weight loss would be (76 – 68 =) 8kg. This would be a sensible target to adopt, realistic and – hopefully – achievable. Having a realistic target is essential.

Other experts have suggested looking at your current weight and then planning to lose perhaps 10% of that over an initial three months; and some have suggested being even more cautious and aiming at losing only 5% of your starting weight over that time. The more gradual the process, the more likely you are to keep the weight off.

How fast should you lose weight?

You should aim to lose your excess slowly but steadily. This is tied in to having a realistic target; if you set yourself a very ambitious one, then you may be tempted to try and shift as much as you can in as little time as possible. This is definitely

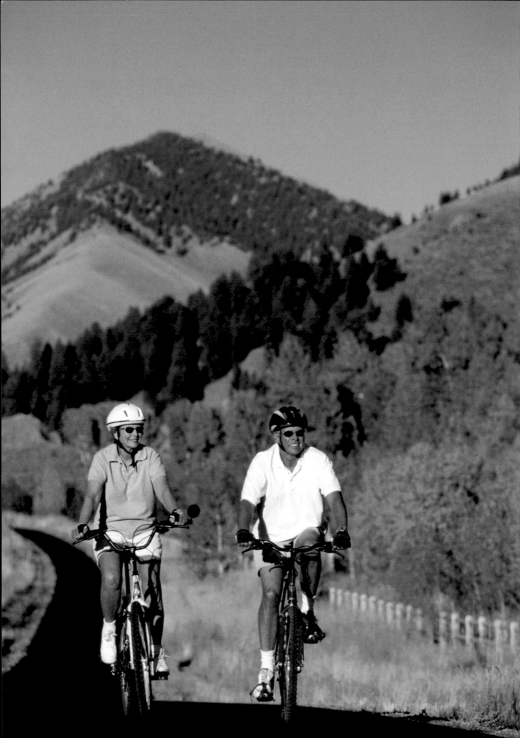

not the best solution, and is the reason why many people swing from losing weight to gaining it, then trying to lose the weight they put back on – and so forth. This is common, and is known as 'yo-yo dieting'.

Why is slow best?

The role of your resting metabolic rate in weight loss was mentioned on page 7. Your metabolism is the reason why change should be gradual. Even when you're doing nothing, your body is doing a lot – blood is circulating, the heart is beating, you are breathing, hormones are being secreted – and it's using energy to keep things going. The rate at which it uses energy is known as your resting metabolic rate (RMR) or basal metabolic rate (BMR).

When you lose weight too quickly there is a corresponding reduction in your RMR, in part because it is related to the amount of lean tissue (like muscle) that you have. Most weight loss comes from fat, but a proportion is non-fat tissue. If you lose weight quickly, the proportion of lean tissue you lose is greater and your body adjusts by dropping your RMR. Your RMR is responsible for burning more calories in your body than exercise, and when it drops you are using fewer calories to keep your basic processes going. Once you start eating 'normally' again, the weight will pile straight back on. Quite simply, you're no longer using up as much energy as you were, so the excess is deposited as fat. You're tempted to start dieting again – and before you know it, you're yo-yoing… This can be very bad for you, both physically and mentally. It actually results in overall weight gain.

must know

Health promotion
Regular physical activity doesn't just help you look better – it also halves the risk of you developing heart disease or having a stroke.

In many slimming clubs and support groups there are often rounds of applause for the people who have lost the most in any particular week, but that shouldn't really be the case. People who lose fast are the people whose diets will stall later, or who will fall onto the yo-yo rollercoaster – not through any fault of their own. But you can step off the ride. Slowly and steadily is the answer – if you want to do the best for your health and keep the weight off. In practical terms it means a bit of patience and taking a long-term view.

Don't try to lose more than a kilo a week. If you have ten kilos to lose, allow at least three months – twelve weeks. If you have 20 kg, then it should be six months, and so on. And these are the minimum lengths of time, remember. Don't be disheartened if it all seems too slow. Many experts agree that to keep the weight off and make a permanent difference, you should aim to lose no more than 5–10% of your starting weight in six months. The important thing is to keep it off.

Exercise

The only sure way to lose weight has been summarised as 'eat less, do more'. As we've seen, eating less isn't entirely straightforward – it's a matter of what you eat too, of eating better and more healthily. But the 'do more' part doesn't need a lot of qualification. Almost all experts – medics, dietitians, nutritionists – agree that when you start dieting, you should also start increasing your level of physical activity – and they all agree that it's essential to be more active if you want to maintain your weight loss long term.

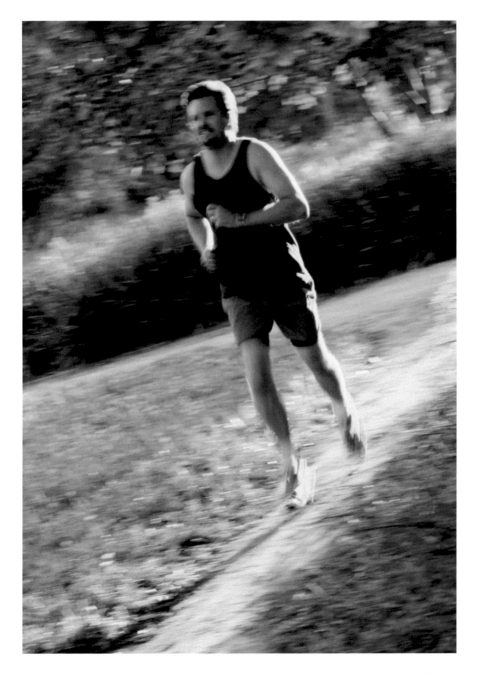

Exercise, especially resistance exercise, helps
your metabolism by building lean muscle tissue, and
that boosts your RMR. Muscle burns more calories
than fat, so once you have increased the amount of
muscle you have you'll be burning more energy,
even when you're sitting still. There's also some
evidence that taking exercise can stabilise blood
sugar levels: exercise, and the amount of muscle in
your body, affects your body's response to insulin in
a helpful, positive way.

Many of us have inactive lifestyles, so the first
thing to do is improve on that, which can be
relatively painless. Increase the level of incidental
exercise you take. Walk to the shops instead of
automatically taking the car, mow the lawn, vacuum
the house – and do those things with a bit of oomph,
get them done quickly. Aim to be more active in
general every single day.

Then you can add extras. Perhaps you might join
a basic exercise class, or take up yoga. If you find the
idea potentially humiliating – and many overweight
people were overweight children who found sport
humiliating at school – then track down an 'exercise
for slimmers' group where everyone's in the same
position. Many public pools run slimmers'
aquarobics, for example, and that can be really
helpful, as exercising in water is much less likely to
result in physical injury. There might even be
women-only sessions: useful if you are female and
embarrassed about being seen in a swimsuit.

Walking is the thing that most people find
easiest to incorporate into their everyday life. Try to
walk energetically; strolling is not the key, though
it's better than driving. Use a pedometer to find out

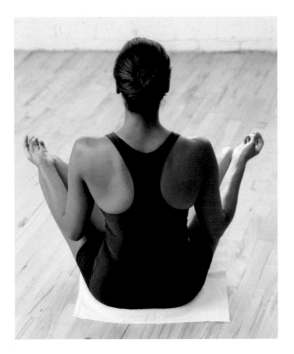

how many steps you take in a normal day, and then build up until you are doing at least 10,000. Several studies have indicated that taking 10,000 steps a day can prevent you gaining weight, even without any major adjustment in your diet. Here are some ideas:

▶ Walk round the block after supper every night

▶ Volunteer to walk a neighbour's dog if you haven't got one of your own, and do so regularly. If you've got a dog, then do the dog walking – and let your pet have an extra walk each day, too.

▶ Pace about when you're on the phone.

▶ Hide the remotes – then you'll need to get up to change the TV channel!

▶ Use stairs whenever you can – gently at first, but build up your stamina until you can actually run from the first to the second floor.

weblinks: www.pedometersuk.co.uk

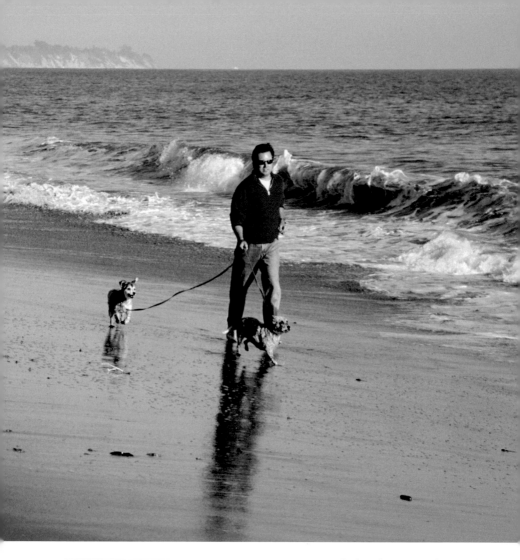

Swimming

Swimming is a great
cardiovascular workout that
targets almost every muscle in
the body while putting hardly
any pressure on the joints.

**Explore the most scenic parts of
your neighbourhood to help keep
motivation high.**

- If you use public transport to travel to work, get off one or two stops before you need to and walk the rest of the way. If you live close enough to work, walk there. If you have to drive, then park further away. Do that at the supermarket too: don't try and get a place near the entrance – park as far away from it as you can.
- Walk up escalators. If you find this impossible without collapsing in a wheezing heap, then build up slowly: start walking two-thirds of the way up, then halfway, then almost at the bottom – then walk all the way.
- At work, walk over to speak to colleagues rather than emailing them; use the loo on a different floor and take the stairs to get there.

Exercise isn't a substitute for dieting. The amount of exercise required to shed just a couple of kilos would be difficult for most people to achieve – for example, a 70kg walker would have to trek for 53km. It is, however, a complement to diet – and it's important for maintaining weight loss. So if you need further encouragement, consider this: the dieters who are most likely to maintain their weight loss are those who have upped their activity levels and made exercise a part of their life.

want to know more?

- If you are obese, enlist some help to get your weight down to healthy levels. Telephone the charity Weight Concern on 020 7679 6636, or visit their website www.weightconcern.com.
- There is sensible general advice at www.weightloss resources.co.uk. It is a membership site, but they have plenty of information that anyone can access without joining.
- Your GP may put you in touch with a slimming group or counsellor if you need some moral support.
- *Collins Gem Calorie Counter* lists the calorie count and nutritional information for hundreds of common foods.
- There's more about different types of exercise in chapter 6, pages 116-23.

must know

Working out calorie needs
For a rough guide to your daily calorie needs, multiply your weight in kilos by 33 if you are a moderately active woman and by 37 if you are a moderately active man. Multiply by 26 if you are a woman leading a largely sedentary lifestyle, and by 31 if you are a sedentary man.

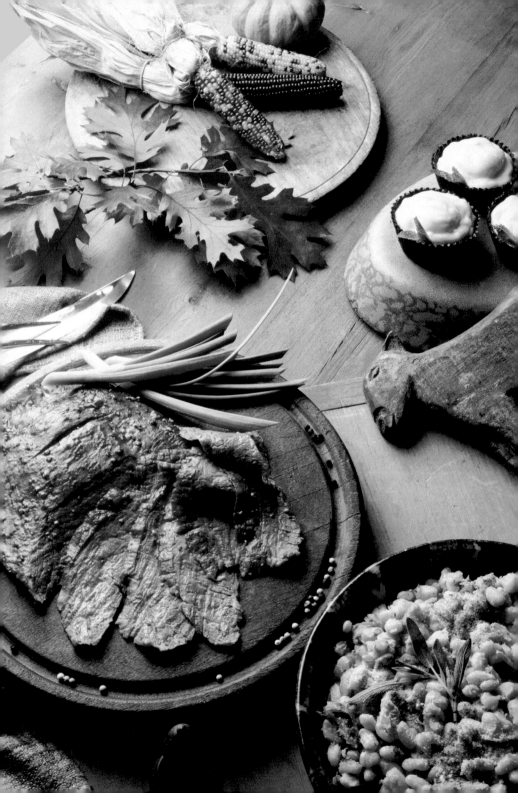

3 Getting started

You understand the logic and like the idea of not having to follow set meal plans, weigh every single ingredient and tot up calorie totals at the end of the day. So what do you do next to get started on the GI+GL diet? Start opting for low GI/GL food choices – it's that simple!

Getting started

Once you know how the GI+GL diet works the practicalities kick in. It's an extremely simple and adaptable diet to follow when you understand the basic principles.

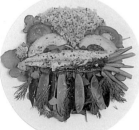

Half veg, quarter protein and no more than a quarter of the plate starchy carbs.

Monitor yourself

Before you start dieting keep a food diary for a week; it's very useful. Write down everything you eat. Everything – even the half biscuit you polish off at the end of a meeting, the last slice of toast that no one else wants. It's a reality check. We don't always realise just how much we're eating, and it can be shocking to look back on later. It's a great exercise to repeat if things seem to drift during your diet. Do you eat more when you're tired? Bored? Stressed? Upset? Premenstrual? Work out your usual patterns.

You must remember this...

There are some more things to think about if you want to lose weight successfully. Firstly, calories do still count. Food only has a GI/GL value if it contains carbs so some really fattening foods, like cheese, don't have one. You'd never lose weight if you ate only carb-free food, but you would make yourself ill. Nor can you avoid fat or protein altogether, for the same reason, so you need to think about how much high-calorie food you're eating. There's no need to break out the calculator, though...

Because the second important thing to remember is that portion size matters. You'll be concentrating on low-GI/GL, low-calorie food, so a few basic guidelines are all that's really necessary – but you have to stick to them. It's not hard. Initially, think of your plate as being divided into quarters. Half should be taken

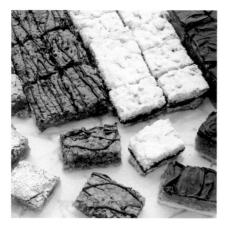 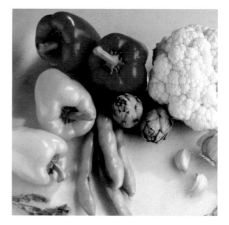

up by vegetables (but not potatoes), a quarter by protein, and no more than a quarter by potato, rice or pasta – the lowest GI version possible, so new potatoes rather than baked, basmati rice rather than ordinary white rice. The essential rule to remember is moderation; use a normal dinner plate, not some gigantic platter! Be firm with yourself; it won't seem like punishment because hunger isn't normally a problem on the GI+GL diet. Don't have enormous servings; just use your common sense.

Looking at the pictures above, it's obvious which foods you should choose on any diet. Chocolate brownies are high GI/GL and have around 300kcal each, while a portion of red pepper strips is low GI/GL and has around 13kcal.

Stages

Dieting isn't only about losing the weight; it's also about maintaining your new weight. So it's useful to think of your diet in two parts: before and after reaching your target weight. In the first part you need to be more careful and a little more strict with yourself.

In Part 1 of your diet, eat mostly those carbs which have a low GI or GL, shown with green dots in the listings in chapter 9. As far as possible, steer clear of the mediums (the yellows) and avoid the high GI or GL foods (red) as completely as you can if you want to lose weight. And if that's not possible sometimes, then try and eat the high GI or GL item with an accompaniment that has a low or negligible GI/GL.

Again, use your common sense. If you can't get out of eating a baked potato without causing a diplomatic incident, have it with lots of low-GI vegetables or a salad with a little balsamic dressing. Yes, butter or cheese would fit into the low or no GI/GL category, but covering your baked potato in cheddar wouldn't help you with your weight loss.

must know

Beans and pulses
Soaking and cooking dried beans and pulses is more economical than using tins, and there is a slight GI advantage too. But keep tinned beans available; having them handy means you can quickly add them to a soup, salad or stew.

Portion sizes

Portion control is most important with the foods that have low or no GI/GL but are high in calories. Try not to exceed these guidelines (they're all single portions).

▶ Meat, fish and poultry: have a piece about the same size as a pocket pack of tissues or a pack of cards – roughly 75–100 g. One chicken breast is just about right.

▶ Rice: two level tablespoons of dry rice gives about 75g when cooked – a mound roughly the same size as a woman's fist. Don't exceed 40g dry rice.

▶ Pasta: again, don't exceed 40g dry weight.

▶ Potatoes: new boiled potatoes are the only realistic option. Stick to 2 or 3 medium potatoes (and resist the temptation to slather them in butter). Try to forget about the existence of chips altogether.

▶ Oil: use olive or rapeseed oil for preference – but no more than a teaspoon. Using non-stick pans helps keep your oil consumption down.

▶ Nuts: don't eat more than 10 at any one time – except pistachios, of which some nutritionists suggest you can eat as many as 30.

▶ Cereals: no more than 60g dry weight. You may even find that quantity too much – an average bowl of muesli is 50g.

▶ Bread: one slice from a medium loaf. Try to buy organic, stoneground wholemeal with a fibre count of at least 2–3g per slice.

▶ Dairy products: your body needs some, but opt for low-fat or no-fat options, and skimmed milk. Watch out for the sugar content in low-fat fruit yoghurts, though. If you are lactose intolerant and rely on soya milk, which does have a GI value as it's made from soya beans, don't buy the sweetened version.

Shopping the GI/GL way

By now you should have a good idea of what to put in your trolley at the supermarket and what to leave on the shelf. Here's a summary.

Yes to:

▶ wholemeal high-fibre bread
▶ fresh and frozen vegetables, except potatoes
▶ fresh fruit
▶ wholegrain cereals and porridge (not easy-cook, though)
▶ dried and tinned beans, pulses, lentils
▶ skimmed milk, low-fat or no-fat yoghurt, other low-fat dairy products
▶ nuts and seeds
▶ basmati rice
▶ wholemeal pasta
▶ lean meat, fish and poultry, tofu

No to:

▶ ready meals and processed food
▶ sugar and sugary foods (read the labels carefully; baked beans tend to be full of sugar, for example)
▶ sweets and chocolate bars
▶ high-fat items like butter, cheese or crisps
▶ white bread
▶ white pasta
▶ white rice, and any easy-cook rice

must know

Visualise your weight loss
If you need any more motivation, try this trick. You've got a realistic assessment of how much weight you need to lose. Get out the weighing scales and pile up the same weight in books or magazines – you might need to do this in stages; even though books are heavy, a 10-kilo pile of paperbacks would soon overbalance. Then load them into carrier bags and haul them around for half an hour – or as long as you can without injuring yourself. The feeling of relief when you finally put them down will help you imagine the huge difference that losing all that weight will make to you.

weblinks: www.food.gov.uk/healthiereating/salt

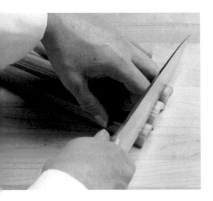

Ideally, you should cook from scratch with fresh ingredients.

Watch convenience foods carefully; we've all got into the habit of using them, and we need to get out of it. Go back to cookery books; many recipes can be easily adapted to work with the GI+GL diet, and there are some tasty examples in chapter 7. When you're shopping watch out, too, for the things you might be doing automatically, like rewarding yourself for being virtuous by sticking a chocolate bar in with the vegetables.

Some food retailers are now listing GI values on their own-brand products. Remember: you're looking out for values lower than 55. Health food shops may stock a wider range of dried beans, organic cereals and healthy breads than your local supermarket, so shop around.

Reading labels

A GI guideline isn't the only thing to look for on food labels; there's a lot of other useful information as well. First, look at the ingredients list. Items are listed according to how much is in the product, with the ingredient with the greatest quantity first – if sugar is listed first, there's more sugar than anything else in the product. Then look at the more detailed nutritional information. Check the:

▶ calorie content, but do remember that the serving size may not be realistic or identical from one brand to another. If you're comparing calorie counts, go for the 'calories per 100g' as a guide instead.

▶ fibre level – high-fibre foods have a lower GI, so look for a minimum of 4g per serving. Always choose the highest, and if you're comparing brands use the 'per 100g' figure.

▶ fat level. Here it's the type of fat that's important. You'll find more information on pages 92–6, but as a general guide avoid foods with a high level of saturated fat or trans fats, which are sometimes called hydrogenated fats. Fat isn't always obvious when you look at the product but it packs a lot of calories, so it's important to check.

▶ salt levels – for your overall health, you ought to look at these too. This is a bit more fiddly as salt is usually given as sodium on labels – you have to multiply by 2.5 to get the quantity of salt. A tin of beans containing 0.8mg of sodium will actually contain 2g of salt – and that's a lot. As a rough guide, 0.5g of sodium per 100g of food is too much salt; less than 0.1g is a little salt. You should think about portion sizes here, too – Marmite has a high salt content per 100g, but you don't eat much of it at one sitting.

Vegetarians are used to reading labels – otherwise they wouldn't necessarily know that some prepared desserts and yoghurts contained animal products (gelatine) – but it's a good habit for everyone to adopt for the sake of their health.

Menus and plans

One of the most important things the GI+GL dieter has to remember is not to skip meals. If there's one thing the GI+GL diet is definitely not, it's a 'how little you can eat' competition. Keeping your blood sugar levels, and therefore your insulin levels, nice and steady is critical to success, so don't be tempted to miss out. This shouldn't be hard, because one of the GI/GL diet's great advantages is its flexibility.

weblinks: www.food.gov.uk/foodlabelling/whatdotheytellme

must know

Nuts
Whenever possible buy nuts in their shells – once they're shelled, they become rancid quickly. If a nut rattles in its shell, it's probably old (except for peanuts, but they're pulses rather than true nuts).

must know

Mind the fat
Be cautious about some foods that are labelled 'fat free' or 'low fat'. It doesn't automatically mean they're low in calories, because they are often high in sugar. Check the full nutritional information.

Porridge

Porridge is a perfect low GI breakfast, but avoid quick-cook or 'easy' porridge. Traditional porridge takes slightly longer to cook – not ages, 10 minutes or so should do it – but it's still got the husks and is high in fibre. It's full of minerals and vitamins, too, and studies have shown that porridge can lower cholesterol levels and so help to prevent heart disease.

Rigid menu plans are often the dieter's downfall; you're missing one vital ingredient or you don't like something you're supposed to eat on day 3, or you just couldn't eat according to the menu plan on day 6 because of other commitments – and there's the perfect excuse for slipping off the diet.

Here are some meal suggestions, which you should treat as mix-and-match rather than rock-hard menu plans. They are guidelines, examples of how you should be eating on the GI+GL diet. They'll give you ideas. You could use them directly, putting them together to suit your life, or use them as a springboard, sparking your own ideas. There are suggestions for snacks, too – up to two a day. Later in the book you'll find more information on specific food types, on getting the overall balance of your diet right, on eating out – and there are some recipes, too. But here's a starting point.

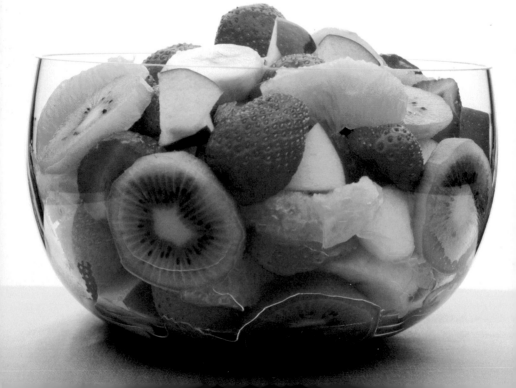

Breakfast

It's vital that you eat a good breakfast. During the night your blood sugar levels will have dropped away, and if you forget breakfast it will be hard to resist snacking later as you try and deal with your body's blood sugar slide. Studies have shown that people who skip breakfast are more likely to be overweight. Make time for it, whatever you're doing; you'll have a better day – and here are some possible choices.

▶ A boiled egg with wholemeal toast
▶ Porridge, made with water or skimmed milk, and served with fresh fruit or a few dried apricots, chopped
▶ Half a grapefruit, a slice of wholemeal toast and Marmite
▶ A one-egg omelette with sliced mushrooms and tomato
▶ Low- or no-fat yoghurt with fresh fruit
▶ Poached smoked haddock with wholemeal toast
▶ A mixture of fresh fruit, dried apricots and a few almonds
▶ Home-made baked beans (haricot beans in a fresh tomato sauce) on wholemeal toast
▶ A home-made yoghurt smoothie
▶ A poached egg on a bed of spinach, with wholemeal toast
▶ Scrambled egg with smoked salmon

Don't be tempted by cereal bars; if you're in a hurry they might seem like a good idea, but mostly they do exactly what they say on the label: they give you an energy boost. That means a sugar spike – just what you are trying to avoid. Making your own fruit smoothie only takes seconds, and the yoghurt lessens the impact of the fruit juice on your blood sugar levels.

Lunch

Many people have to eat lunch out, relying on a sandwich bar or a packed lunch. If you can, choose the packed lunch

Opposite: Fruit salad is a delicious breakfast but for more energy to get you through the morning, pile it on top of a high-fibre breakfast cereal, with a few nuts and seeds and some natural, low-fat yoghurt.

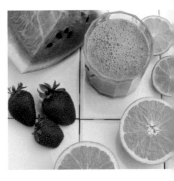

must know

Smoothies

Make your own fruit smoothies – use low fat natural yoghurt and whatever fruit you fancy and whizz them up together in a blender or food processor. If you throw a handful of frozen berries into the blender instead of fresh fruit, you get a ready-chilled one.

because you control what you eat and can avoid pitfalls like high-calorie mayo in a sandwich filling or temptations like treats by the till. And packed lunches don't necessarily have to mean sandwiches, of course. If you feel that you would really miss one, then confine yourself to a sandwich a week, made with wholemeal bread and a healthy filling. Try using hummus or mustard instead of butter. Wholemeal pitta bread is an option, too, and can easily be warmed up in a microwave or toaster (eject it before it actually toasts, though). Many of these suggestions could be included in a packed lunch.

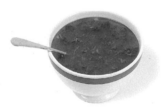

must know

Watch your portions
Don't forget to keep an eye on your portion sizes. You don't have to weigh every single thing; just bear in mind the guidelines on page 46.

Salads – keep them substantial but within GI/GL guidelines, and use lemon juice or vinegar and a little olive oil for dressings:
▶ Salade Niçoise (see page 135)
▶ Tabbouleh (see page 134) with half a wholemeal pitta
▶ Tuna and bean salad (see page 130)
▶ Lentil, chicken and spring onion salad
▶ Hummus (see page 132), with raw vegetable crudités to dip in it
▶ Tomato, avocado and cold roast chicken salad with olives
▶ Greek salad (Horiatiki salata, see page 133)
If you opt for a salad as a packed lunch, then take the dressing separately to avoid it going soggy by lunchtime.

Soups – again, substantial and preferably home-made, because that way you control the contents. Keep them within GI guidelines, which means not thickening them with potato. These shouldn't need it:
▶ Italian chickpea soup (see page 126)
▶ Bean soup (see pages 128 or 129)
▶ Lentil and mushroom soup (see page 127)

You'd have to eat a huge amount of vegetable crudités before you even approached the calorie content of a tuna mayonnaise sandwich.

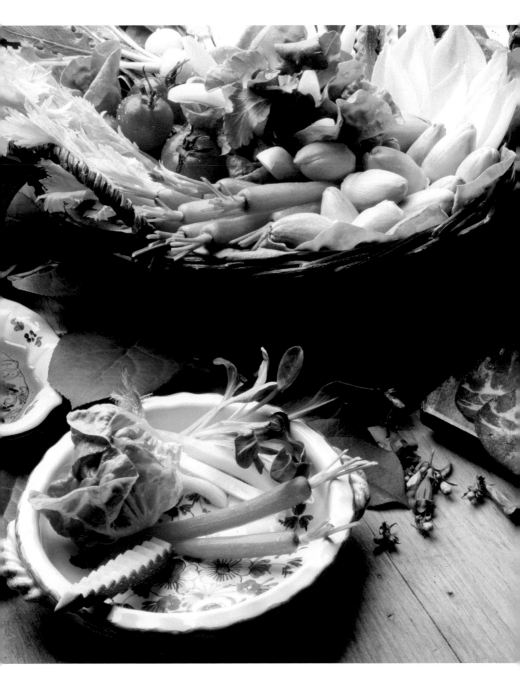

must know

Dried fruits
Dried apricots have
the lowest GI of all
the dried fruits,
and it's worth
buying organic
ones (you won't
need to eat many),
as pesticides can
become
concentrated in
dried fruit.

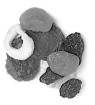

▶ Fresh tomato soup (not creamed, and add some fresh basil)
▶ Spinach and lentil soup – cook them with a little tomato purée
   and black pepper, and blend them roughly.
▶ French onion soup (without cheese and croûtons)

If it's possible to cook a meal for yourself at lunchtime, try a
spinach omelette with a green salad, Thai noodles with
beansprouts and tofu... there are lots of possibilities. And if you
want something sweet after your lunch, go for a piece of fruit or
a low-fat yoghurt.

Snacks

You won't feel the same gnawing hunger on a GI/GL diet as you
might on others, but it's still useful to have something to tide
you over – remember, avoiding plunges and spikes in your blood
sugar level is essential. Here are some suitable stopgaps. Don't
have more than two of these a day, whenever you need them –
maybe mid-afternoon and before bed.

▶ crudités with a small dollop of hummus
▶ 4 dried apricots
▶ an apple or orange
▶ 16 olives
▶ a small pot of natural low-fat yoghurt with fresh fruit
▶ low-fat cottage cheese with raw vegetables
▶ 10 almonds
▶ a handful of berries, cherries or grapes
▶ 30 pistachios
▶ an oatcake spread with low-fat cream cheese

Dinner

The vital thing to remember with the 'main' meal of the day is
portion control – a quarter of your plate filled with protein, a
quarter with rice, pasta or potatoes, and a half with other
vegetables. With meat, make sure you buy lean cuts and avoid

processed meat products (sausages, pies, haggis, black pudding). Take the skin off chicken and turkey, and never use breaded or battered fish or seafood. Fried food is out in most cases – though stir-frying, for example, can be done using very little oil. Eat as many vegetables (except potatoes) as you want. You can go wild with salad, too, but watch dressings. A few suggestions:

► chicken roasted with rosemary and lemon
► chilli beans (see page 143) with a slice of wholemeal bread and a green salad
► chicken kebabs with oven-roasted vegetables
► courgette and tomato dhal (see page 138)
► salmon herb packets (see page 145) with mixed vegetables
► chilli con carne
► chicken curry (see page 140) with basmati rice and salad
► grilled fish with spring onions, ginger and soy sauce
► wholewheat spaghetti with fresh tomato sauce and a salad...

must know

Open top
Turn ordinary sandwiches into open sandwiches – just take off the top slice of bread.

Stuff lemon quarters inside a chicken and sprinkle with herbs.

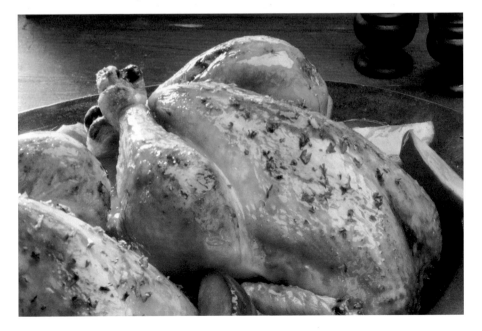

3 Getting started

must know

Making kebabs
Marinate the meat for extra flavour: pieces of chicken can go into a mixture of lemon juice, garlic and a little olive oil for about an hour before being threaded onto skewers, and yoghurt is good with lamb. Several hours beforehand, cut lean lamb into cubes and mix it with low-fat natural yoghurt, lemon juice and a teaspoon of olive oil. Don't forget vegetables: put chopped onion, peppers, mushrooms – whatever you fancy – in a sealable plastic bag with a little olive oil. Close the bag and shake it gently but thoroughly, coating the pieces. Skewer them and grill, but without using more oil.

Over to you! Many recipes can be adapted to the GI+GL diet, and those from some parts of the world – Greece, for instance – hardly need adapting, though you may need to reduce the quantity of oil, or substitute olive oil for other types. That shouldn't affect the overall recipe too much.

Desserts are a bit more difficult as they tend to be high in sugar and fat. If you are prepared to use sugar substitutes you may be able to adapt existing recipes, but generally it's better to go for fruit (watch some dried fruits) and use low- or no-fat natural yoghurt instead of cream. Be inventive with fruit

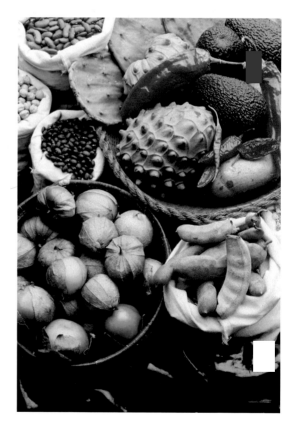

Choose unusual fruits in the supermarket and discover new favourites.

salads – theme them by colour, or try tropical fruits – and use a couple of teaspoons of Cointreau instead of a sugar syrup (especially good with strawberries).

Convenience foods and ready meals

There's been an extraordinary growth in convenience food in recent years, which has been linked directly to the rise in obesity. Whatever the role of ready meals, they aren't a great idea on the GI+GL diet. Many are high in fat and salt, have unexpected ingredients and preservatives, and often don't contain enough vegetables or fruit. They can be unsatisfying and the suggested portion sizes are often small – an alleged meal for two is frequently more like a realistic meal for one (and that means that the nutritional information – calorie count, etc – which you considered carefully is now inaccurate, as you'll eat double). They're a minefield.

Use your freezer to stock up on meals that can be heated in a hurry. When you make a freezeable dish like a chicken curry (see the recipe on page 140), for instance, make extra portions and freeze them in microwaveable freezer containers for your own, low GI/GL, perfectly healthy ready meals. Frozen vegetables are another useful convenience food; keep a supply in your freezer and you'll always have them to hand.

want to know more?

▶ See the recipes in chapter 7 for some simple, tasty low GI/GL dishes.
▶ For more recipes, see *Antony Worrall Thompson's GI Diet*, 2005.
▶ The Tesco website www.tesco.com gives GI ratings for many of their products, including some ready meals, and they also give GI ratings on the packaging of own-brand products.
▶ Much of the information for diabetics is useful for GI/GL dieters too. Check out the advice on adapting recipes in Diabetes UK's website www.diabetes.org.uk/eatwell
▶ See chapter 8 for advice on eating out in restaurants and fast food joints, and chapter 9 for the GI/GL ratings of some common foods.

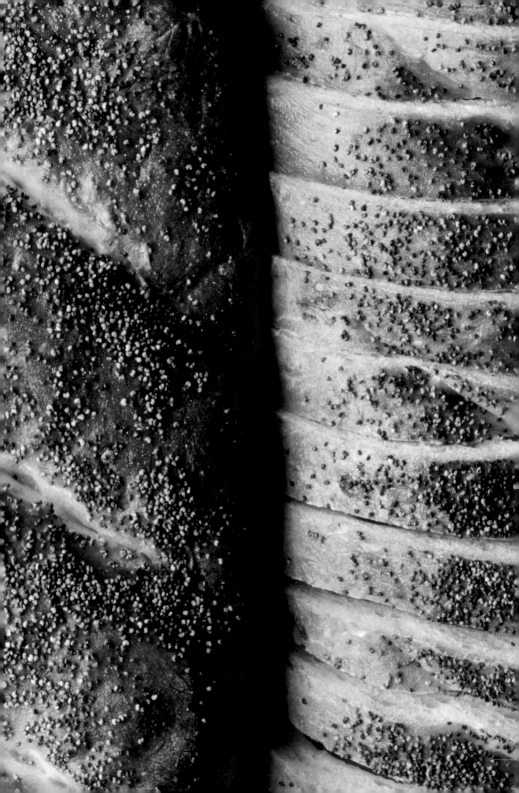

4 Food and drink

You know the general GI/GL rules, so now it's time to get more specific. Which type of rice should you choose, and what kind of bread? Are some fruits and vegetables better than others, and are any banned or restricted? How can you use low GI/GL ingredients to put together nutritious meals? This chapter explains the guidelines for each type of food and drink.

Food and drink

Flexibility is one of the major advantages of the GI+GL diet, but it is important to understand how your food and drink affects you in order to make the best choices.

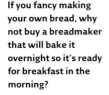

Types of food

In this chapter you'll find essential information and suggestions about particular categories of food, arranged alphabetically, and then some about drink, both alcoholic and non-alcoholic.

Bread, baking and biscuits

The kind of bread and cereals you eat is the single most important factor in the overall GI/GL of your diet. You need to choose products which are slow to be digested and absorbed by your body. Some diet gurus tell dieters to avoid bread altogether, but for many of us this is unrealistic; it's an important part of our diet. Go for a grainy bread, with at least 3g of fibre per slice, and look for stoneground wholemeal bread and flour. Stoneground is more coarsely ground and has other advantages over flour made in roller mills (as most is these days) – not only is it a great source of fibre, but it also contains B vitamins and some of the minerals your body needs. Even so, you will still need to watch the quantity you consume. Pumpernickel, sourdough and rye breads (those without lots of wheat flour) are all possibilities, too. Definitely avoid all kinds of white bread – ciabatta, baguettes, sandwich bread, even 'fortified' white bread – as your body breaks it down very rapidly.

Go for stoneground wholemeal flour in any home baking too, and avoid white flour. Gram flour (sometimes used in Indian cooking) is made from chickpeas and so has a lower GI than wheat flour. Wholemeal pastry affects blood sugar more slowly than other types, and savoury ingredients, especially

If you fancy making your own bread, why not buy a breadmaker that will bake it overnight so it's ready for breakfast in the morning?

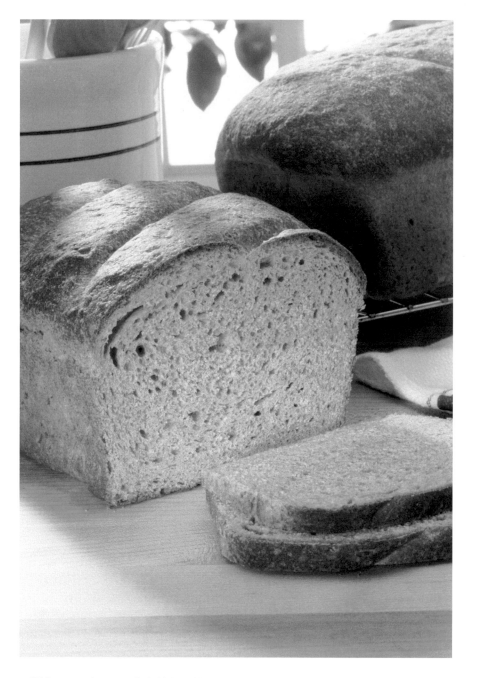

must know

Clean your beans
Before soaking any dried beans
or pulses pick them over and
discard any stones or grit. Most
are 'recleaned' in the UK, but it's
as well to be sure.

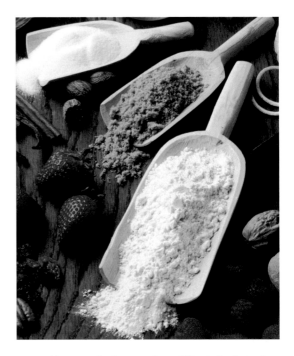

**Bake with wholemeal flour and
keep sugar to a minimum. Dried
fruits will lower the GI/GL value
of a cake or loaf.**

vegetables, are the best options. Watch for fattening
quiche or pie contents, like cheese – but it's best to
avoid pastry altogether, if you can.

Sweet biscuits don't belong on any diet, let alone
a GI+GL one. Savoury ones, like oatcakes, are better
but check the label for fat content and go for those
made with olive rather than palm oil. Then read the
fibre levels and opt for the oatcakes with the highest
fibre count (probably 'rough' rather than 'smooth').

As far as other bakery products go, remember
that they'll all produce a blood sugar surge – and
that includes those croissants, Danish pastries and
savoury pasties too. You may quell a temporary
feeling of hunger, but the satiated feeling won't last,
and you won't be doing your diet any good in calorie
terms, either.

Beans and pulses

Beans and pulses are an excellent source of protein and fibre – calcium, potassium, magnesium, iron and B vitamins, too – and most are low GI/GL. They are an easy way of reducing overall GI levels; adding them to soups, casseroles, and salads will slow down your digestion. Beans are also probiotics, keeping the digestive system itself healthy.

There are many different kinds and they can be used in many different ways, so if you don't care for one just try another. Dried beans can be kept almost indefinitely, though they shouldn't be; old beans take ages to cook, for one thing. Some dried beans need to be soaked overnight, while others need only a few hours and lentils shouldn't need soaking at all. Once your beans have been soaked, drain off the soaking water and boil them in fresh water for about 10 minutes before simmering them until they're tender. A few tips:

▶ Don't cook beans in their soaking water
▶ Don't add salt to the cooking water
▶ Always rinse canned beans before heating them or adding them to your cooking.

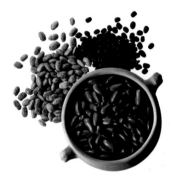

Try some of the more unusual types of beans – like anasazi, black turtle, fava, great northern, lima or navy beans.

You can freeze soaked and cooked beans in batches, and they'll keep for several days in the fridge if they're covered well. Canned beans are a valuable standby, so keep some in your cupboards; there are some excellent bean mixtures available which are great for salads. Watch out for tinned baked beans – the sauce they are in is often high in calories, containing lots of fat and often sugar, too.

Lentils – brown, green, 'Le Puy', orange, yellow – are particularly rich in protein, fibre and B vitamins.

weblinks: www.bestlowcarbs.com

Diabetics have found lentils useful as your blood sugar levels remain stable no matter how many you eat. They do, however, have a fairly bland, slightly earthy flavour and are best cooked with onions, spices and herbs, and garlic. They're ideal for thickening soup, make a delicious accompaniment to grilled meat and fish and are an essential ingredient in many Indian recipes. Wash and sort them – checking for any little stones – before cooking.

Breakfast cereals

The importance of having breakfast can't be overstated, but it is essential to make a sensible choice. If you're considering cereals then you can't do better than porridge: it can be varied with fresh fruits, chopped dried apricots, pumpkin and sunflower seeds, a few nuts, low-fat natural yoghurt... and will see you through to lunchtime. Otherwise, opt for cereals containing bran or oats, but without any added sugar. Go for those with the highest fibre count and avoid quick-cook porridge or instant oats completely.

Butter, fats and oils

We all need fat in our diet, even when we're trying to lose weight, because essential nutrients are supplied by 'good' fats. Those are the ones you should choose and that means, essentially, using olive or rapeseed oil and avoiding trans fats and saturated fats that come from animal products (such as butter). Don't buy oils in huge quantities as flavours can go off if they are left too long.

Try to cut back on the amount of fats you use, even of the 'good' fats. Buy an oil sprayer and use it with your olive or rapeseed oil; it will help you use much less. You could also buy ready-mixed spray oils which are generally a mixture of oil and water, though check what sort of oils they contain. Making your

Opt for grains with their husks still on.

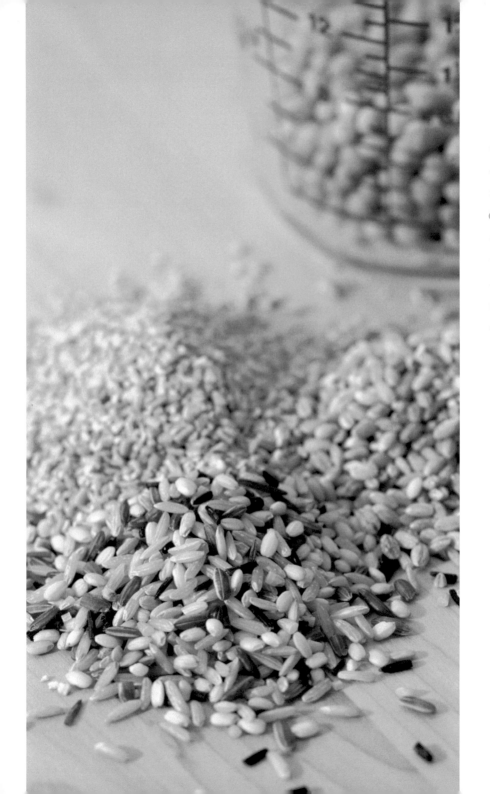

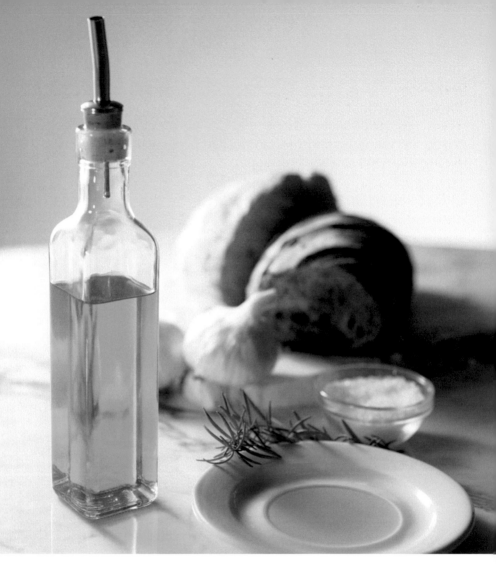

Dip your bread in a little olive oil instead of slathering it with butter.

own mix to use in your sprayer is easy: go for 1 part of oil to 7 parts of water. Use reduced-fat dairy products for yourself, but don't give them to children under 5, who need the full-fat versions. Try making salad dressings with low-fat natural yoghurt instead of olive oil.

There's more information about 'good' and 'bad' fats on pages 92–6.

Dairy foods

Most dairy products don't have a GI or GL rating because they don't contain carbs, and don't therefore affect blood sugar levels. Milk and yoghurt, however, contain natural sugars. Choose low-fat versions of all dairy products because although they have no or low GI/GL values, they contain high levels of fat – and saturated fats too, which could raise cholesterol levels and clog up your arteries.

One thing you shouldn't do is try and eliminate dairy products from your diet (see pages 102-3 for advice for vegans). They are an important source of calcium, which is vital for the health of your bones, and the EC official recommendation is that we all get 1,500mg of calcium a day. If you aren't getting enough in your diet, then your body will use the calcium in your bones to enable it to function. This may lead to osteoporosis and other bone-related disorders. Two to three servings of low-fat dairy products should give you sufficient calcium.

Some people are lactose intolerant. Lactose (a sugar present in milk) isn't found in yoghurt or cheese, so you could opt for them instead, or look for foods fortified with calcium, like high-calcium soya milk. Dried figs are another good source, as are

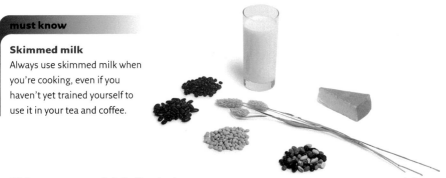

must know

Skimmed milk
Always use skimmed milk when you're cooking, even if you haven't yet trained yourself to use it in your tea and coffee.

green leafy vegetables (especially broccoli), tinned salmon or anchovies (eat the bones) and eggs.

Eggs

Eggs are carb-free, but do contain cholesterol. Because of this some nutritionists recommend that you avoid eating eggs or consider only using the whites. Pregnant women are advised to be wary of uncooked eggs because of the risk of some infections. However, eggs are a valuable source of vitamin E, and it is possible to buy them enriched with omega-3 fatty acids (see below). Don't fry them; boil or poach them in Part 1 of your diet. In Part 2, omelettes can be cooked in a non-stick pan that has been sprayed with a little oil.

Fish and seafood

Fish doesn't have a GI because it's not a source of carbohydrate. Oily fish (mackerel, herrings, salmon and the like) are an excellent source of omega-3 fatty acids which have many benefits – reducing blood cholesterol, calming irregular heartbeats and boosting your immune system – and are thought to play a part in the treatment of depression and Alzheimer's disease. All fish is a good source of protein, and eating more has been linked to a significantly diminished risk of having a fatal heart attack. Shellfish contain cholesterol (see pages 93–4), so should be used infrequently, and any fish coated in batter or breadcrumbs should be avoided completely, as should those which come with a sauce based on flour.

must know

Canned fish
Choose fish canned in mineral water or brine rather than oil, then rinse it before you eat it. One US study found that 76% of the salt added to canned tuna was removed by rinsing it.

Torpedo-shaped fish like salmon or mackerel have more healthy oils than flat fish like plaice or sole.

Fruit

Always eat fruit whole and unpeeled – the extra fibre from the skin will help slow the absorption of fructose, the naturally occurring fruit sugar. Don't drink juice instead as it's much, much more quickly absorbed by your system. To demonstrate how fast this is, diabetics who have a hypo – a collapse due to low blood sugar – are often given orange juice, as it is the fastest way of getting glucose into the bloodstream.

Not all fruit is low in GI value. As a broad indication, tropical fruits – like pineapples and paw paws – tend to have a higher GI than others. At the other end of the scale, most berry fruits are difficult to test accurately as they contain such a small amount of carbohydrate. Fruit is a source of antioxidants (see pages 96-8) which have a powerful protective effect on the immune system – they are associated with reduced levels of heart disease and also of some cancers.

Jams and marmalades

Sadly, most of these contain high levels of sugar. If you can't wean yourself off them completely, use those which contain extra fruit and reduced sugar. Try the brands designed for diabetics or visit your local health food shop and find some alternatives. Even if you make your own, and can restrict the quantity of sugar you use, it still won't have a low GI. In GL terms, though, a little is permissible – most are medium GL – but make sure you keep to a teaspoonful. It doesn't take long to get used to savoury spreads instead, but watch peanut butter (and other nut butters) as they're very high in calories. Marmite is an excellent choice because of its high vitamin B content.

Meat and poultry

There are no GI levels for meat or poultry unless it has been processed. Watch out for calorie levels, trim off any visible fat and always remove chicken or turkey skin. Serving size is crucial

must know

Sauces for fish
If you like a creamy sauce with fish or shellfish then substitute a fresh tomato salsa with a bit of chilli in it. It is so different and refreshing that you won't miss your mayo or hollandaise. It works as an alternative to ketchup, too.

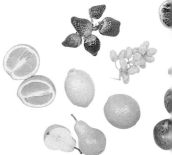

Eat at least two portions of fruit a day, choosing ones with different colours.

Fruit spreads

Check out fruit spreads. These are often surprisingly low in calories compared to jams and can be used on top of porridge, for example. But do check their ingredients and don't use any spread where the first listed ingredient is sugar. Remember: on labels, the greatest quantity comes first.

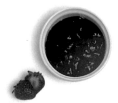

Pot-roast meat with water or stock, herbs and vegetables, rather than roasting in oil.

and you need to consider overall portion control. If you are used to eating huge amounts of meat, don't worry – you'll soon adapt to eating less, and you won't need it to bulk out your diet anyway. Grilling any red meat, which naturally contains fat, is the best option for anyone following a weight-loss programme; frying would just add more calories.

Many people are concerned about the welfare of animals raised in modern farming conditions, and the quantities of antibiotics and growth hormones that can be administered to them. If this bothers you, choose organic meat and poultry; the extra cost won't seem so horrific when you are consuming less on your GI+GL diet.

Nuts and seeds

Watching quantities is really important here as nuts are very high in calories, though they are often recommended as a GI/GL-friendly snack. They are a principle source of 'good' fat, essential to our overall health, and contain significant amounts of vitamin E and selenium, so don't avoid them entirely – just limit your intake.

Almonds are a great choice. Peanuts aren't actually nuts; they're legumes like peas or beans, and develop underground as their alternative name – groundnut – suggests. Avoid salted peanuts and opt for the dry roasted variety instead. Sunflower and pumpkin seeds are packed with vitamins and minerals, and make a good alternative snack to nuts. They can also be used as salad ingredients: dry-roast them in a frying pan (using no oil) until they begin to colour and then scatter them on top of mixed salad leaves.

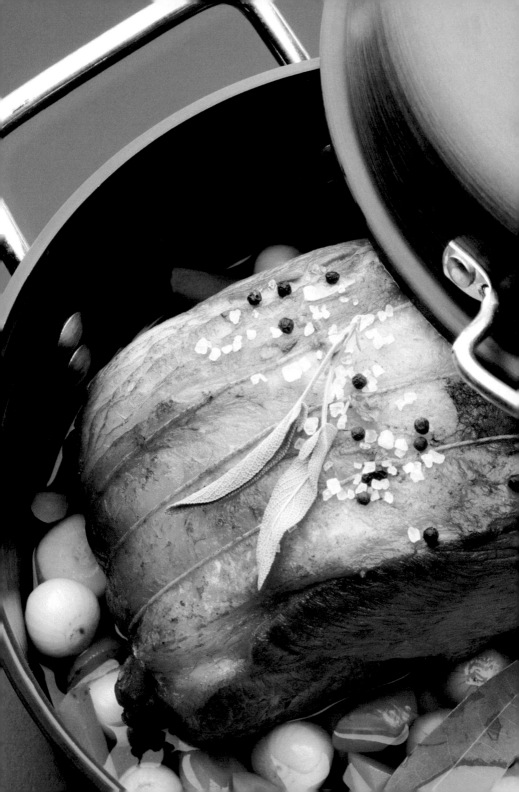

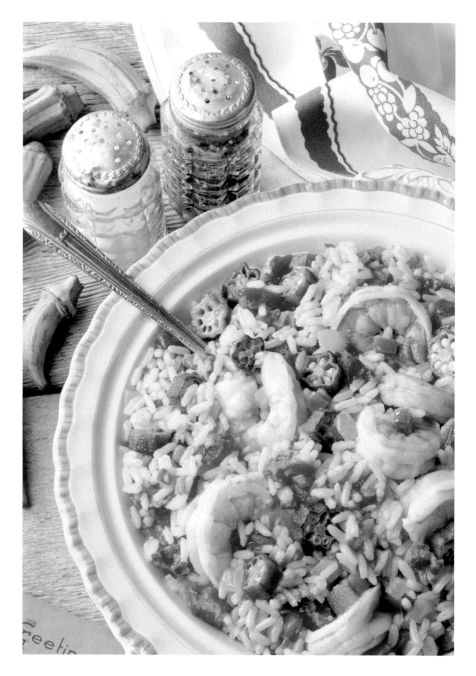

Pasta

Pasta has a reasonable GI value but a high GL, meaning that an average portion would have an undesirable effect on blood sugar levels. Keep the portion size small, remembering the plate portion control trick, and try to eat pasta as a side dish, not the main focus of the meal. Canned spaghetti has a higher GI, and the sauce will inevitably be full of sugar and salt. If you are a pasta-lover, use the following guidelines:

▶ Choose wholemeal pasta. If you find one brand too heavy, then try another.
▶ Combine pasta with a low-GI sauce and add vegetables. Cheese-based sauces are too high in calories, and often thickened with flour. Lay off the Parmesan – it's quite a high-fat cheese.
▶ Avoid ready-made pasta sauces – cook your own using fresh ingredients.
▶ Egg pasta and filled pastas, like spinach and ricotta stuffed tortelloni, have a lower GL than some of the other kinds but they have a higher fat content, so bear this in mind.
▶ Take pasta off the heat while it's still *al dente* – with a bite to it.

Include plenty of vegetables in rice dishes to lower the overall GI/GL value of the meal.

Rice and noodles

Basmati rice, brown rice and long-grain rice are all medium GI, largely because of the type of starch they contain – amylose – which is broken down in the digestion more slowly than others, but it's still high GL because of the average portion size. Don't overcook your rice or you'll raise the GI. Avoid easy-cook rice of any kind, or the sticky rice that often goes with Chinese or Thai food. Risotto is usually made with arborio rice, which releases starch during cooking and therefore has a high GI: the starch granules have swollen and burst, and are digested quickly. Noodles aren't a great alternative, as rice noodles are high GI and wheat noodles are medium. Cellophane noodles, which are made from mung bean flour, are the best choice.

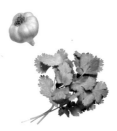

Use natural flavourings like
garlic and herbs.

If you make your own
chutneys and pickles, you
can control the sugar
content.

Sauces and pickles

Many ready-made ones are high in flour and sugar
and should be avoided. Home-made is best, but
there are still potential pitfalls. Don't, for example,
thicken gravy with flour; just serve some of the meat
juices with a teaspoonful of wine or sherry added to
the roasting tin instead. Here are some other tips.

▶ Mint sauce is simple. Chop a handful of mint
leaves and cover with a tablespoon of white wine
vinegar, then add a little sugar (or you could use
sweetener).

▶ Unsweetened apple purée is a great substitute for
bottled apple sauce

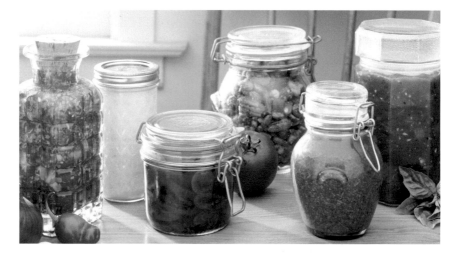

▶ To make your own tomato ketchup, blend finely
chopped tomatoes, red pepper, red onion and
garlic with cider vinegar and a little sugar, and
store it in the fridge.

▶ Salad dressings should always be home-made; use
twice as much oil as vinegar and add things like
crushed garlic, herbs and mustard as flavourings.

Put all the ingredients into an empty, clean jam jar with a securely fitting lid and shake them together vigorously.

Sugar and sweeteners

Sugar has no nutritional benefits as such: no vitamins, no minerals, no protein, nor any other nutrient. It's just calories and should be avoided as much as possible on any weight-loss diet, not just a GI/GL one, largely because it can be difficult to use in moderation. In addition, it's in so many processed foods that it can be quite hard to work out how much you're actually eating. It is vital to check the ingredients lists on labels for sugar as it appears in many, often unpredictable, foods.

Having said that, sugar shouldn't be completely criminalised: one study showed that people who ate a lot of bread over time put on more weight than those who ate sweets. It's the quantity. Use a little if you want, and if you feel you can stop at that.

If you use sugar in tea or coffee, gradually cut it back. Many scientists are worried about artificial sweeteners, especially aspartame. If you're trying to wean yourself off sugar, try using fructose, a natural fruit sugar. It has a lower GI than ordinary granulated sugar and it's also sweeter, so you'll need less. You can use fructose in home baking, but bear in mind that it is much sweeter and that it cooks at a lower temperature. Most packs of fructose have clear guidelines on use.

As with everything else, moderation is the key. If you like sugar and eat a lot of it you will find it hard to lose weight. When you cut down, your body will adapt and you will be healthier for it.

must know

Soups

Lower the GI value of homemade soups by adding whole ingredients like pearl barley, lentils or beans. And when you liquidise or blend a soup, only blend half – add the rest unblended and mix them together. This helps by giving your digestive system more work to do, and adds an interesting contrast in texture, too.

weblinks: www.www.holisticmed.com/aspartame

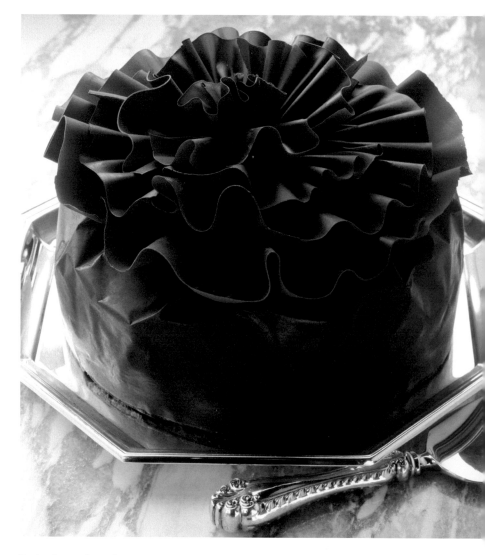

During Part 2 of your diet, you could allow yourself a small piece of cake under the 80:20 rule. Just make sure you stick to low GI/GL foods for the rest of the day.

Sweets and chocolate

Following on from sugar, most sweets really are out... it's so hard to stop at one. The exception, and only really for Part 2 of your diet once you have reached your target weight, is dark chocolate with at least 70% cocoa solids. Most chocolate contains large amounts of saturated fat and sugar, but in high-cocoa chocolate there is much less. It is also rich and delicious, so you don't need much – never eat more than 20g in any one day (that's about a fifth of a standard bar). Go for a piece of fruit or a couple of dried apricots if you get a sweet craving; like all cravings, it will diminish as your body adapts.

Vegetables

An almost completely green-light area. Even those vegetables with a high GI (like broad beans) usually have a low GL once portion size is taken into consideration. There are a few exceptions, notably potatoes and other starchy root vegetables – parsnips, beetroot – which should be eaten in moderation, as should winter squashes. As a broad guideline, vegetables containing a lot of water like spinach, salad leaves, onions and courgettes have the lowest GI. Carrots, tomatoes and peas are slightly higher but also contain valuable nutrients. Sweet potatoes have a lower GI than ordinary potatoes and can be cooked in the same way – boiled, mashed or baked. Canned vegetables tend to lose vitamin C during processing but frozen ones usually retain their vitamins and minerals better.

Buying organic can make a huge difference to the taste of vegetables, and you will avoid the pesticide residues found in non-organic produce.

must know

Chocolate berries
Gently melt 70% chocolate in a bowl over a pan of simmering water. Dip strawberries or cherries into it and leave them to cool – a spectacular after-dinner treat. It's a fun way to get children involved and enjoying healthy eating.

must know

Where are they from?
The sooner that fruit and vegetables are eaten after picking, the more nutrients they contain. Imported produce can take ages to arrive in the UK, so 'Produce of...' is another thing to remember while checking labels.

If you grow your own, try to be as organic as you can. You don't even have to have a garden; many varieties work well in window boxes. Salad leaves are good to grow and most suppliers sell packs of mixed leaf seeds; if you cut the baby leaves regularly, more will keep coming up. In fact, you don't even need a window box to grow your own; you can buy windowsill lettuce – small plants in pots – in many large supermarkets.

Bean sprouts only need a jam jar to grow in – and you can vary the varieties. Use a large jar and a clean fine cloth. Soak whatever seeds you want to use – try alfalfa, or lentils – in water overnight. Pop them in the jar and cover the open jar with the cloth (a rubber band will hold it in place well). Rinse and drain them by tipping the jar, so the water passes through the cloth, twice a day. Keep them in a dark place and they should be ready to eat in three days – give them some sunlight before use.

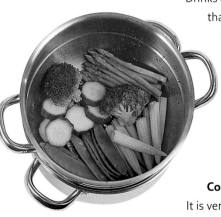

Steam vegetables lightly to retain the vitamin content.

Types of drink

Drinks are deceptive. We have a tendency to assume that a drink is somehow lower in calories than a solid food – but a simple milkshake from a major fast-food outlet can actually contain more calories than an entire meal. Never forget to think about what you're drinking as well as what you're eating. In the following pages, we'll look at non-alcoholic drinks first, then get on to the hard stuff.

Cold soft drinks

It is very important to keep your level of hydration up. Most nutrition advisers recommend that you drink at least six to eight glasses of still water every day. Don't be tempted to flavour your water with fruit squashes or cordials, or drink fruit

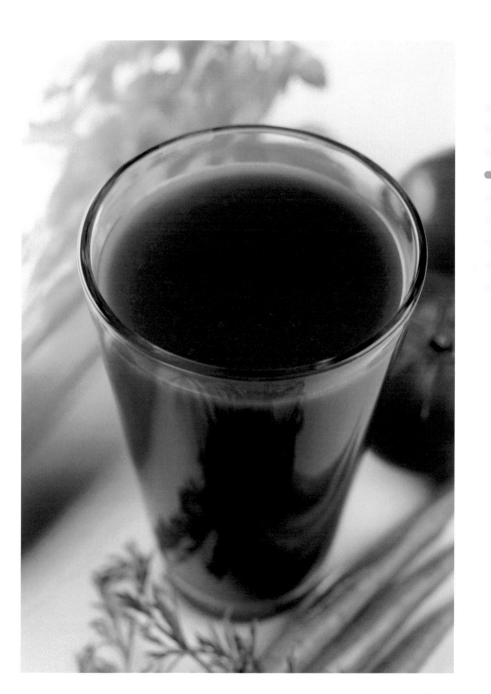

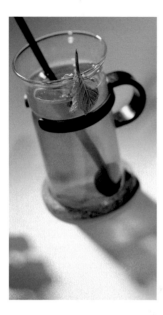

Some herb teas have medicinal benefits. Peppermint tea is a good *digestif* after a meal.

juice instead of water – they all affect your blood sugar levels swiftly. Drinks with a cola base are particularly bad; not only do they contain sugar and/or artificial sweeteners, they also contain significant amounts of caffeine, which is very bad for your insulin levels (see below). The best choice is water, still, with no fancy additives.

Hot drinks

Some dietitians recommend that you only drink decaffeinated coffee and tea because caffeine leads to increased insulin production. Monitor your caffeine intake and cut down if it's excessive – more than four or five cups a day. Real espresso, made the Italian way using high-pressure steam, is not as harmful as you might suppose because the steam causes the flavour to be released in a concentrated form, without releasing too much caffeine at the same time.

Tea has less caffeine than coffee. It also contains antioxidants (see pages 96–9) which are good for your heart and circulation, and may help to prevent the development of some cancers; in fact, there are more antioxidants in tea than in any vegetable so far tested. You can drink more tea than coffee without it seriously affecting your diet.

If you are not already a fan of herbal teas, it's well worth giving them a try; you may be pleasantly surprised by the delicious flavours available. Some are supposed to have health benefits, too: peppermint and nettle are good for the digestion; camomile and verbena are relaxing; and lemon balm can lift your mood... Great things have been claimed for green teas, and they certainly have high levels of antioxidants. Jasmine tea, the classic green tea used in Chinese restaurants, is easy to find and very refreshing. Squeeze your tea bag – you'll release twice as many of the antioxidants.

Drinking gallons of coffee to wake you up, and perhaps munching a chocolate biscuit on the side, will have the opposite effect to the one you want. Drinks which contain caffeine, when combined with the rapidly absorbed sugar in sweets, biscuits and chocolate, encourage your body to produce adrenaline. Sounds as though it might be effective, but adrenaline causes blood sugar levels to rise, giving only a short-term boost followed swiftly by the inevitable plunge. Adrenaline is a stress hormone, and too much of it can make you moody and irritable. You should find that you no longer need your coffee to wake you up when you're on the GI+GL diet. You shouldn't start to flag in mid-morning or afternoon, because eating in accordance with GI/GL guidelines will keep your blood sugar levels steady all day long.

Alcohol

Most diets recommend avoiding alcohol altogether during the first phase, when you are trying to get down to your target weight, and the GI+GL diet is no exception. But that's in an ideal world, and many people find it very difficult not to drink at all. Moderation, moderation, moderation is the only key to success. It's best to think of alcohol as an occasional indulgence when you're trying to lose weight. It doesn't have any nutritional benefits to make up for all the calories it contains, though some health benefits have been claimed for red wine.

weblinks: www.alcoholconcern.co.uk

> **must know**
>
> **Coffee detox**
> If you normally drink a lot of coffee and want to reduce your caffeine intake, cut back gradually rather than just stopping. This will help prevent withdrawal symptoms like headaches and irritability. A good way of cutting down almost imperceptibly is to switch to using a smaller cup.

A glass of red wine a day may lower your risk of heart disease – but more than two a day increases it.

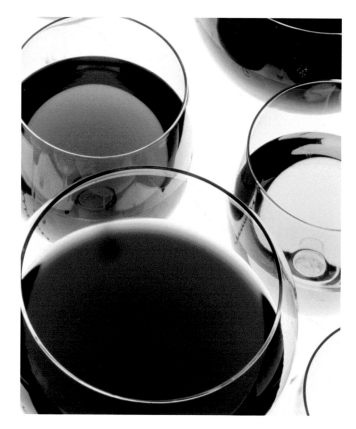

Alcohol is digested in the stomach, so it enters the blood stream quickly. This results in increased insulin production, plummeting blood sugar levels and the need for something to push those levels back up – food... or more alcohol. And with more alcohol goes every good dieting intention. If you can't settle for only drinking a little alcohol (and you'll know if you can't), then it is best to eliminate it completely. Reintroduce it, in reduced quantities if you drank a lot, once you have reached your target. If your weight starts to increase again, cut the amount of alcohol back. A painless way of reducing the amount of wine you drink is to change to smaller glasses; use the standard pub measure – 125 ml – glasses instead of larger ones.

Alcohol actually prevents you from losing weight. Really. The form of energy provided by alcohol is very easily utilised by the body, and while this is happening it doesn't need to use its fat reserves as a source. The impact is much higher when the stomach is empty, so if you do decide to drink alcohol then make sure you always have it with a meal to minimise the rate of absorption.

If you can compromise, go for dry wines, preferably red because of the health benefits, and avoid sweeter wines, beer, lager and stout. Beer has a high GI because it contains maltose, an extremely high GI sugar. If you are tempted by beer it might help you to remember that 'beer bellies' weren't given that name for nothing. Although drinking a lot of any type of alcohol will cause you to lay down excess abdominal fat, beer is one of the worst offenders. The evidence is that excess belly fat is an active, living part of your body. The protein and fatty acid combination the fat generates causes cells to proliferate – something directly linked to the development of cancer tumours. If you've got a beer belly, don't fool yourself: there's no doubt about the fact that it's damaging your health. Try not to drink beer at all in the first part of your diet, and afterwards make it a rare treat.

There are recommended safe drinking limits – between 21 and 28 units per week (3–4 per day) for a man, and between 14 and 21 units per week (2–3 per day) for a woman. These are maximum limits and even if you drank the lower quantities you would still be consuming a lot of empty calories. If you are trying to lose weight, don't drink more than 7 units a week, and be careful about increasing that as you try to maintain your weight; be prepared to drop back. One unit of alcohol is:

▶ 125 ml (a standard pub glass) of wine
▶ 300 ml (half a pint) of beer or lager
▶ 50 ml (a pub measure) of sherry, aperitif or liqueur
▶ 25 ml (a pub measure) of spirits.

must know

Alcohol calories
What's your tipple? A 500ml can of bitter contains 160 kcal, while 500ml of dry cider has 180. A 125ml glass of wine will have between 85 and 120 kcal. Whisky and ginger ale – 165. Gin and tonic – 184. A small coffee liqueur – 80. Now multiply by how many you drink in an evening.

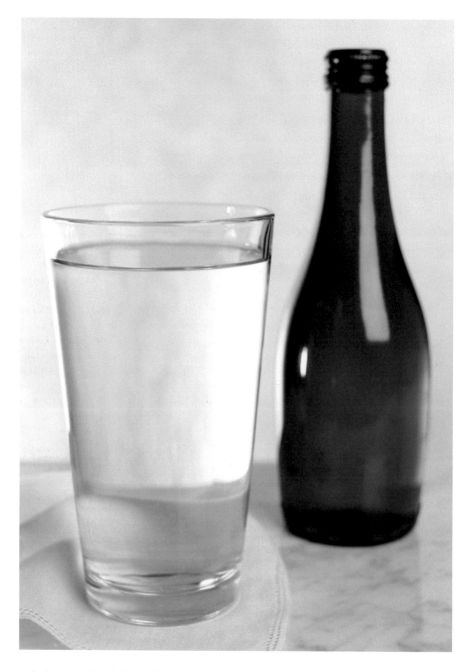

There's been some debate about whether alcohol used in cooking – in a stew, like the cassoulet with cod in the Recipe chapter (see page 141) – actually retains any alcohol. The best answer so far is 'almost certainly not'. If the stew is prepared normally, the alcohol will evaporate, leaving the flavour behind. And a little can be useful in other circumstances: using a small amount of Cointreau, for instance, on a fruit salad is a permissible alternative to using loads of sugar syrup. If you don't want to use alcohol, then try sprinkling a little orange flower water (available in most health food shops) instead.

Don't forget... drink

One final thing on drinking: don't forget to do it! We all need liquid, but not lots of caffeine-loaded hot or cold drinks, or alcohol. When you are busy it is easy to forget the need to drink and some people seem to confuse the sensations of thirst and hunger, leading them to eat when their body really needs liquid.

Dehydration doesn't just increase the chance of you overeating; it causes an increased loss of concentration, more headaches and dropping energy levels. If you know you are going to be involved in an activity where it will be difficult to get a drink, or where you might forget, then take a bottle of water with you. Remember your six to eight glasses a day.

want to know more?

► If you suspect you might have a drink problem, contact Alcoholics Anonymous on 0845 7697555 to be put in touch with your local branch.
► If you're interested in finding out more about how to protect yourself from heart disease, visit the Coronary Prevention Group website (www.healthnet.org.uk) or telephone 020 7927 2125.
► You can also contact the British Heart Foundation on 020 7935 0185, www.bhf.org.uk.
► See chapter 5 for advice on how to balance the different nutritional groups in your diet.
► See chapter 7 for low GI/GL recipes, chapter 8 for advice on eating out and chapter 9 for the GI/GL ratings of some common foods.

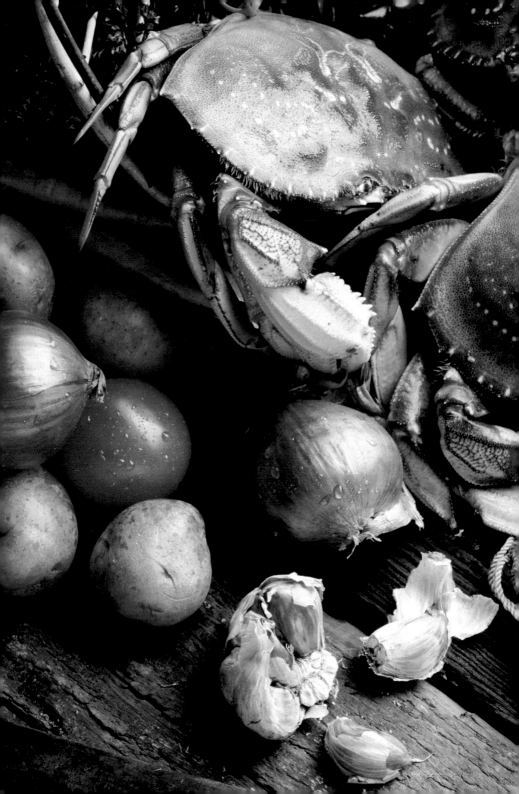

5 Balancing your diet

You could eat exactly the same low GI/GL foods day in, day out and, sure enough, the weight would start dropping off. But you wouldn't be getting all the nutrients you need for optimum health and before long you could start suffering the symptoms of a vitamin or mineral deficiency. There's no point in being slim but ill, so read through this chapter to find out what your diet needs to include.

Balancing your diet

Our bodies need to obtain certain nutrients from food in order to function efficiently, so the overall balance of your diet is vitally important for your health, not just your weight loss.

must know

Portion sizes
When using the Food Pyramid, keep the serving sizes to the portions described on page 46.

The GI food pyramid

The GI+GL diet has met with such a favourable reaction from medics and dietitians because, if you follow it properly, it provides a balanced diet. And once you are beyond the weight-loss stage, its aim is to keep you eating in a fully balanced way for life. We couldn't survive long term on a diet that excluded whole food groups like fats or carbs, despite what some diet gurus might have you believe. The trick is to consume each food group in the correct quantities relative to each other. The GI food pyramid below shows the different types of food and their recommended daily servings.

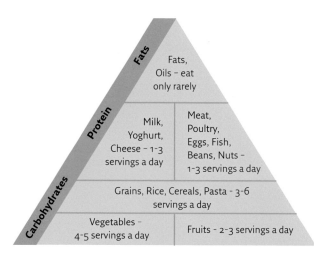

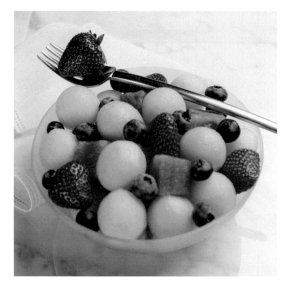

Devise your own multi-coloured fruit salad combinations.

Carbohydrates

The World Health Organisation recommends that we eat 400g of fruit and/or vegetables every day for optimal health, which is the basis for the UK's 'eat five a day' campaign. Five fruits and vegetables each day should provide both the recommended daily levels of fibre and the minimum amounts of all the vitamins and minerals we all need.

Eating more fruit and veg than this has been linked with reducing the incidence of minor colds and flu, as well as lessening the risk of more serious conditions like heart disease and some types of cancer. It can lower cholesterol and reduce the risk of strokes, asthma and even cataracts. However, surveys show that most people don't even manage to get their 'five a day'. This may be partly due to some confusion about what constitutes a portion. Here are some guidelines:

- ► half a large fruit, like a grapefruit
- ► one medium-sized fruit, like an apple or orange
- ► two small fruits, such as plums or apricots
- ► a slice of pineapple, melon or mango
- ► a teacupful of small fruits like grapes, berries or cherries
- ► a tablespoon of dried apricots (or dates or sultanas, but watch their GI and note that dried fruits only count as one portion, no matter how many you eat in a day)
- ► three tablespoons of sieved, puréed or tinned fruit (avoid tinned fruits in thick sugar syrup – super-high GI/GL)
- ► a dessert-size bowl of salad
- ► two tablespoons of cooked vegetables
- ► and pulses, like lentils, beans (and peas) only count as one portion no matter how much you eat during the day.

Potatoes don't count at all; nor do plantains or green bananas, which are considered to be starchy carbs for this purpose.

Vegetables have slightly more health benefits than fruit, so try and eat more of them. However, the really important thing is to get lots of variety. A quick way of doing that is to eat fruit and veg of as many different colours as possible. The UK's Stroke Association has been

Make vegetables the basis of your meal, and serve with a small portion of protein.

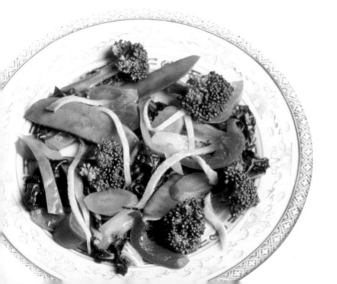

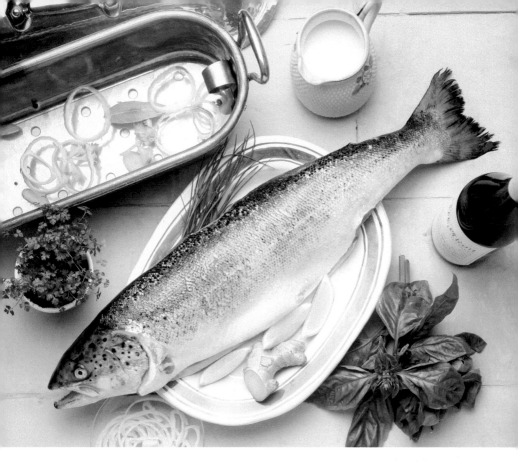

campaigning for an improved diet under the 'eat a rainbow' slogan – it's a snappy line, easy to remember, and relevant to everyone, young and old.

Eating fewer starchy carbs – potatoes, pasta, rice and bread – does seem to bring health benefits, not simply in terms of reduced weight and the positive consequences of that. You'll feel the benefits quite quickly if you cut back on grain-based carbs, potatoes and sugar.

Proteins

Most people in the developed world eat more than enough protein, and too much can be bad for the kidneys. Ever-increasing portion sizes in restaurants don't help. When we think of protein we automatically think of animal sources, but it

Use a fish kettle to steam fish and you'll retain more of the nutrients.

must know

Raw vegetables make a great snack, especially when dipped into home-made hummus. See page 132 for a recipe.

comes from vegetable sources too – beans, pulses, tofu and nuts. Animal sources tend to be higher in saturated fats and studies with diabetics have illustrated the consequence of this: people who obtained most of their protein from plant rather than animal sources had lower blood cholesterol – and better blood sugar control – than those who ate mostly animal-derived protein. This doesn't mean that you have to stop eating meat, but it does indicate that you should vary your meals and make some of them vegetarian.

Proteins are made from amino acids, many of which are essential to our health. Vegetable-based proteins can be deficient in one or more of these amino acids, but by combining them you can get the right balance. Hummus is a great example: it mixes chickpeas and tahini – sesame seed paste. So is the masoor dhal with courgettes and tomatoes in the Recipe chapter (see pages 138-9) when combined with a chapati (see page 151); serving it with a cucumber raita would also add an excellent source of calcium. Brown rice and beans are complementary proteins, as are wholegrain cereal and milk. There's more advice for vegetarians on page 102.

Fats

We need some fat for our bodies to function. Unfortunately most of us eat too much fat, and fat of the wrong kind. And many of us get confused: cholesterol is a fat, and if cholesterol is bad for you, for example, how come eating some foods high in cholesterol can be good? Here's some guidance on types of fats, starting with the ones that are best for you.

Monounsaturated fats

Found in olive, groundnut and rapeseed oils, spreads made from those oils, and walnuts and avocados. These have a beneficial effect on the heart.

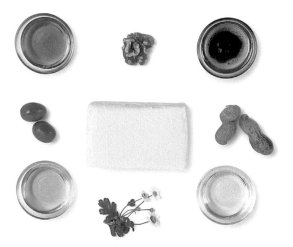

It's not always easy to judge the type of oil or fat in a product. Read labels carefully.

Omega-3 polyunsaturated fats

Found in cold-water fish like mackerel, herring, salmon, tuna and sardines; in linseed, wheatgerm, sesame seed, soya beans, the eggs of grain-fed chickens and in evening primrose oil; also in olive and rapeseed oils. These help to thin the blood and are essential for brain function.

Omega-6 polyunsaturated fats

Found in vegetable, sunflower and corn oils, soya margarines and sunflower spreads. They don't have all the health benefits of omega-3 fats but they're still better than saturated fats and trans fats. They have the same high calorie levels as other fats, so use them sparingly.

Saturated fats

Found in animal fats – lard, butter, suet, meats (including poultry skin), dairy products, eggs – and in coconut, palm and palm-kernel oils. They're often used in processed foods, like biscuits, pies and crisps. A lot of saturated fat in the diet can raise your level of cholesterol, a type of fat in the blood.

> **must know**
>
> **Cooking oils**
> Read the labels carefully, because some oils will decompose if heated – extra virgin olive oils, for example. Use them for salad dressings instead. Store all oils in a cool, dark place and don't keep them for longer than three months, as they can go off.

weblinks: www.www.omega-3info.com

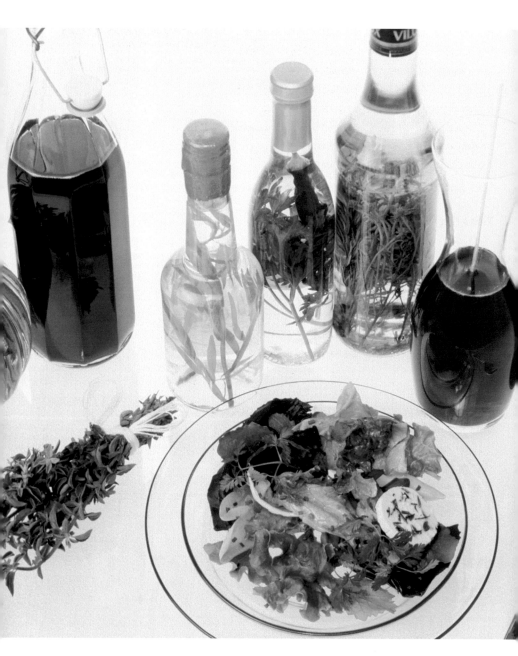

There are two types of cholesterol – HDL is the beneficial kind and LDL is dangerous. High levels of LDL can clog your arteries with fatty deposits, making it harder for blood to circulate and increasing your risk of heart attack and stroke. Cutting back on saturated fats and opting for heart-healthy foods can stabilise and even lower your blood cholesterol count and increase your life expectancy.

Try flavouring salad oils with fresh herbs, garlic or chillies.

Trans fats or hydrogenated fats

The worst kind, linked to high cholesterol levels and increased rates of heart disease. They are often by-products of hydrogenation (hence their alternative name), a process used to make unsaturated fats firmer and more spreadable. They're found in biscuits, cakes, some spreads and margarines, breads and fast foods. They can also lurk in surprising places, like cereal bars, so check the labels. The UK's Soil Association has banned their use, and anything bearing the SA's organic symbol will be fine. Many manufacturers are trying to cut the levels of trans fats in their products and you should try and eliminate them completely from your diet for the sake of your health.

A good move is to cut down on fat intake all round – which will help you to lose weight. Then you should look at reducing the quantity of saturated fat in your diet and replacing it with omega-3 essential fatty acids, which are actually good for us. Monounsaturates are the best; they lower bad, LDL cholesterol and are thought to increase the proportion of good, HDL cholesterol in the blood.

must know

Healthy oils
Choose cold-pressed oils and try some different types as well as olive oil: rapeseed, sesame, soybean, flaxseed and canola oils are all healthy. See if you like the flavours.

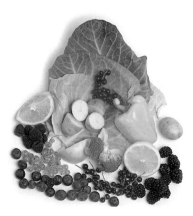

Remember to 'eat a rainbow' every day to get a wide enough range of micronutrients.

Research has shown that the dietary cholesterol present in eggs, seafood and offal actually has a lesser effect on your blood cholesterol than eating saturated fats. If you already have a blood disorder then you will probably need to avoid dietary cholesterol completely, but for most people cutting down on red meats, butter and cheese is the critical thing. Just be moderate in your use of seafood, offal (if you like it) and eggs.

When insulin levels are high, the level of HDL – good – cholesterol is reduced and evidence is beginning to emerge that eating low GI/GL food can lower the effect of 'bad' LDL cholesterol. This is yet another reason to follow a GI+GL diet which aims to regulate your insulin levels.

Vitamins and minerals

A balanced diet isn't just a matter of carbs, protein and fats. We also need a range of vitamins and minerals. Most of us can get these from a properly balanced diet, but we do need to give it some thought. The chart opposite will give you a guide – make sure that you are eating foods containing each vitamin and mineral on at least a weekly basis.

Antioxidants

Antioxidants have had a lot of favourable publicity recently. They are thought to be protective, since they 'mop up' a lot of the free radicals present in the body. Free radicals are by-products of normal bodily processes, which cause some of the problems associated with ageing, but they can be exacerbated by pollution, cigarette smoke, illness or exposure to ultraviolet light. Numerous studies have shown that

Vitamins and minerals

Vitamin A Eggs, butter, fish oils, dark green and yellow fruits and vegetables, liver.
Essential for: strong bones, good eyesight, healthy skin, healing.

Vitamin B1 (Thiamine): Plant and animal foods, especially wholegrain products, brown rice, seafood and beans.
Essential for: growth, nerve function, conversion of blood sugar into energy.

Vitamin B2 (Riboflavin): Milk and dairy produce, green leafy vegetables, liver, kidneys, yeast.
Essential for: cell growth and reproduction, energy production.

Vitamin B3 (Niacin): Meats, fish and poultry, wholegrains, peanuts and avocados.
Essential for: digestion, energy, the nervous system.

Vitamin B5 (Pantothenic acid): Organ meats, fish, eggs, chicken, nuts and wholegrain cereals.
Essential for: strengthening immunity and fighting infections, healing wounds.

Vitamin B6 (Pyridoxine): Meat, eggs, wholegrains, yeast, cabbage, melon, molasses.
Essential for: the production of new cells, a healthy immune system, production of antibodies and white blood cells.

Vitamin B12 (Cyanocobalamin): Fish, dairy produce, beef, pork, lamb, organ meats, eggs and milk.
Essential for: energy and concentration, production of red blood cells, growth in children.

Vitamin C Fresh fruit and vegetables, potatoes, leafy herbs and berries.
Essential for: healthy skin, bones, muscles, healing, eyesight and protection from viruses.

Vitamin D Milk and dairy produce, eggs, oily fish.
Essential for: healthy teeth and bones, vital for growth.

Vitamin E Nuts, seeds, eggs, milk, wholegrains, leafy vegetables, avocados and soya.
Essential for: absorption of iron and essential fatty acids, slowing the ageing process, increasing fertility.

Vitamin K Green vegetables, milk products, apricots, wholegrains, cod liver oil.
Essential for: blood clotting.

Calcium Dairy produce, leafy green vegetables, salmon, nuts, root vegetables, tofu.
Essential for: strong bones and teeth, hormones and muscles, blood clotting and the regulation of blood pressure.

Iron Liver, kidney, cocoa powder, dark chocolate, shellfish, pulses, dark green vegetables, egg yolks, red meat, beans, molasses.
Essential for: supply of oxygen to the cells and healthy immune system.

Magnesium Brown rice, soya beans, nuts, wholegrains, bitter chocolate, legumes.
Essential for: transmission of nerve impulses, development of bones, growth and repair of cells.

Potassium Avocados, leafy green vegetables, bananas, fruit and vegetable juices, potatoes and nuts.
Essential for: maintaining water balance, nerve and muscle function.

Selenium Brazil nuts, fish, whole grains, garlic, mushrooms, broccoli, cabbage, onions.
Essential for: normal cell growth, regulation of hormones, protection against cancer and immunity from infections like colds and flu.

must know

Think chunky
The more work your body has to
do in order to digest food, the
better. Think whole grains,
chunky rather than puréed
soups, fruit rather than fruit
juice. It will soon become
automatic.

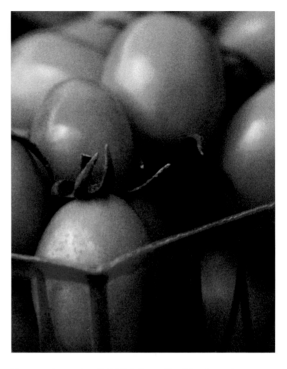

**Tomatoes contain the antioxidant
lycopene which protects against
some cancers, especially prostate,
colon and stomach.**

those who eat a diet high in antioxidants reduce
their risk of getting heart disease, several types of
cancer and cataracts.

Antioxidants are found in fruit and vegetables
and include the essential vitamins A, C and E.
Lycopene, found in tomatoes, is another valuable
antioxidant; it becomes more effective when the
tomatoes are cooked or processed, so canned
tomatoes are a great addition to the diet. Tea
contains antioxidants called flavonoids – and green
tea is thought to be particularly high in them.
Selenium is another significant antioxidant, and
Brazil nuts are a good source. Eating in accordance
with GI/GL guidelines should ensure that your diet
has enough of these powerful substances.

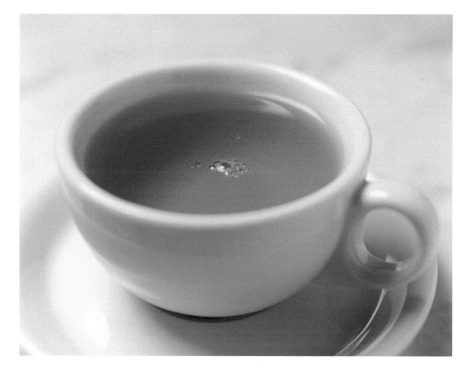

Salt

Eating too much salt is associated with hypertension (abnormally high blood pressure), and high blood pressure increases your risk of having a serious heart condition or a stroke. Not only does too much salt cause hypertension, but some researchers also believe that persistently eating too much salt can have a more harmful effect on your health than taking up smoking. According to them, it will take twice as many years off your life.

For the sake of your health, the UK government has recommended that your total daily salt intake – including the salt in processed foods – should be a maximum of 6g. This is equivalent to just over a level teaspoon but, on average, the majority of

It is said that tea was invented in China in 2737 BC when leaves from a camellia bush fell into the emperor's cup of hot water.

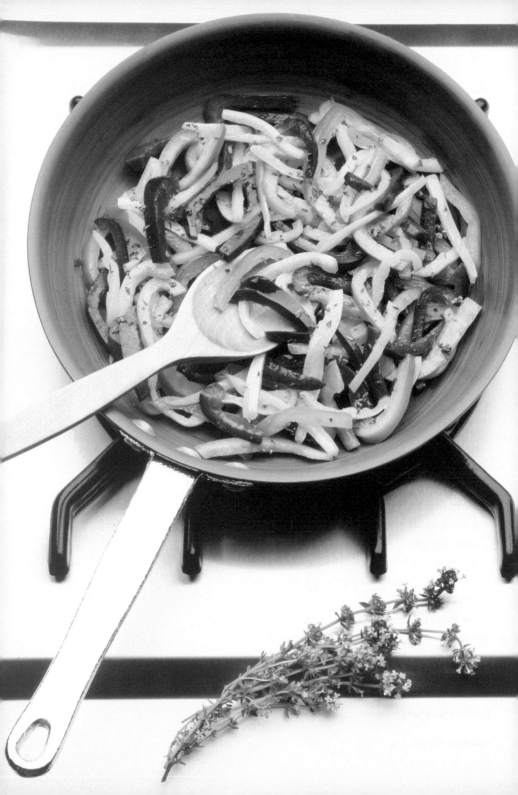

people in the UK consume nearly double that – most of it from manufactured food. Restricting or avoiding processed foods will help to ensure that you eat a more balanced diet all round. It will also reduce the amount of salt and sugar you eat. Only about a third of our excessive salt intake is added in cooking or at the table. Cutting down can only benefit your health, so here are some tips.

► Watch those processed or manufactured foods; avoid them whenever possible.
► Read food labels very carefully. Salt is shown as sodium and you have to multiply that by 2.5 to get the amount of salt. Ideally look for less than 0.1g of sodium.
► Cut down on all salty foods: crisps, savoury biscuits, salted nuts. Cured and smoked foods like bacon, sausages, smoked and canned fish are also very high in salt while fresh foods have only a small amount.
► Reduce the quantity of salt you use in cooking. A recipe that serves four should contain no more than half a teaspoon of salt.
► Never add salt at the table.
► Experiment with herbs and spices as alternatives. Black pepper is particularly useful, and the flavour that other spices and herbs impart to a dish can compensate for a lack of salt.

There are salt substitutes on the market but be careful – they contain potassium and shouldn't be used by anyone with kidney problems. As with sugar, your taste buds will adjust to lower levels over time, and you'll come to prefer less salty foods. It may not take long.

Sprinkle fresh or dried herbs on your stir-fries to enhance the flavour.

must know

Don't be fooled
Nutritional information on packaging can be deceptive. 'Fat-free' means the product has less than 0.15 g fat per 100g, but '90% fat-free' means it has 10% fat. 'Virtually fat-free' means it has less than 0.3g of fat per 100g; 'low fat' means it has to have 3g or less per 100g. 'Reduced fat' means it contains 25% less fat than the standard equivalent.
'No added sugar' means that sugar hasn't been added during manufacture; it doesn't mean that the product contains no sugar at all. And 'unsweetened' means that no sugar or sweetener has been added. 'Reduced salt' has, as yet, no legal definition. The Food Standards Agency recommends that anything so labelled should have 25% less salt than a normal equivalent.

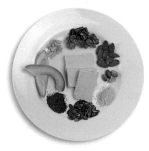

Vegetarians need to educate themselves about protein sources that will provide them with all the essential amino acids.

When pregnant, women need twice as much iron.

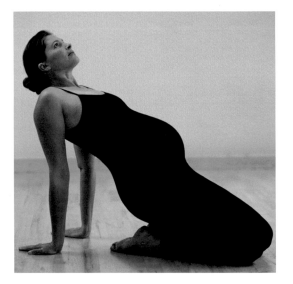

The GI+GL diet and vegetarians

Vegetarians have a head start with the GI+GL diet as they tend to use more low GI/GL foods, like pulses and nuts, anyway. If you're vegetarian you risk not getting enough iron, needed for the transport of oxygen in the blood, because red meat is the prime source. Most vegetarians are quite aware of this and take measures to ensure they get the iron they need, like eating more pulses or nuts and supplementing their diet with vitamin C, which aids the absorption of the form of iron found in plant sources.

If you are vegetarian and need to lose weight then start by checking the amount of nuts you use. You may also have got into the habit of using a lot of cheese, and vegetarian cheese – made without animal rennet – is often high in calories, so watch that too. Check fat and calorie levels carefully. The other thing that you might be doing is eating too much bread. Keeping a food diary will help you work out where the excess calories are creeping in.

Some vegetarians use soya protein (or tofu) as an alternative to meat, and many doctors believe that everyone, vegetarian or not, should eat at least 25g of soya protein a day anyway, because of its health benefits. It is low in carbs and saturated fats, and contains an excellent range of B vitamins, calcium and iron. You can increase the amount of tofu you eat relatively easily – add cubes to vegetable kebabs or casseroles, for example. If you use soya milk, which has a lower GI than rice milk and is therefore a better choice in GI/GL terms, go for unsweetened – but select a brand that contains added calcium.

If you are vegan, the GI+GL diet should present few problems. You'll need to take a vitamin B12 supplement, as this vitamin normally occurs in meat, fish, eggs and milk; it's also present in yeast. You should also monitor your calcium levels carefully (see box, right).

must know

Calcium
Calcium isn't just found in milk products. Non-dairy sources include green leafy vegetables, dried fruit and the sort of oily fish where you eat the bones, like anchovies, canned salmon or sardines.

The GI+GL diet in pregnancy

Pregnancy is not the time to think about weight loss, but it is the time – possibly the most important time – to make sure you are eating healthily. If you are pregnant and thinking about losing weight, you must talk to your doctor. He or she may recommend that you change to a healthier form of eating but don't, whatever you do, try to stick to Part 1 of the GI+GL diet, the pre-target-weight plan. Good nutrition is crucial both to your health and the health of your baby. You need to be as fit as you can, while not using pregnancy as a reason for overeating. Following GI/GL guidelines within a balanced diet is a smart choice.

There are some specific nutrients to consider. Pregnant women, and those who are breastfeeding, must make sure they have enough protein. You also need a diet rich in iron, and one that includes vitamin B6 and folic acid – eating spinach, Brussels sprouts, cauliflower, broccoli, cabbage and beans will help. Oranges are full of vitamin C and that aids

must know

Full-fat milk
Children should not be given semi-skimmed milk before they are two – and then only if they are eating a varied diet. They shouldn't be given skimmed milk at all if they're under five.

the absorption of iron. Your intake of calcium has to be kept up, too – it's important for forming your baby's bones and teeth, while looking after yours. Many pregnant women take a specially designed vitamin and mineral supplement during pregnancy, and this can be a good idea.

Cut sugary foods, preservatives, salt, saturated fats and trans fats, and processed and refined foods. Some doctors think you should avoid alcohol completely when pregnant, while others advise that you stick to two or three drinks a week. Drink plenty of plain water, though; this is especially important when you are breastfeeding.

The GI+GL diet and children

Obesity in childhood has increased a lot in recent years, but different body mass index guidelines apply to anyone under 18, so consult your doctor before putting a child or young person on a diet. They're still growing and their bodies are still developing, so a nutritionally complete diet is essential. Children's weight can sometimes be deceptive; they often seem to increase in size just before a growth spurt, so be aware of this.

As the GI+GL diet is essentially a way of eating sensibly, its guidelines are useful. Don't apply those specifically for weight loss – just guide children away from high-sugar, high-saturated fat options and towards lower GI/GL foods. Getting them accustomed to eating healthily will give them lifelong benefits, so it is definitely worth doing.

Ensure they always eat breakfast (though not high-sugar cereals), have a good lunch and dinner and eat appropriate snacks – if they are full enough

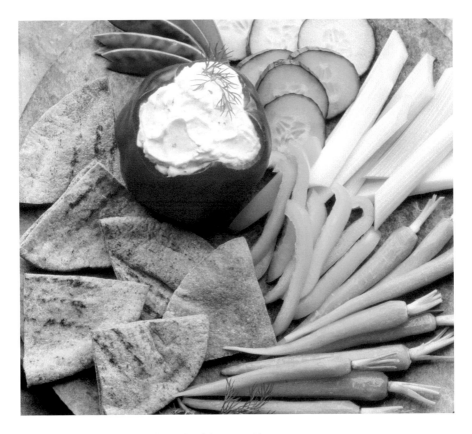

they won't be too tempted by unhealthy ones. If you bring them up to eat vegetables from the start you (probably) won't have so many fights about them.

Vegetable strips, pitta bread and dips make an ideal light lunch for children.

Don't give children low-fat products; they're still growing and need enough fat in their diets – but 'good' fat, not saturated fat or trans fats. Encourage them to be active instead of collapsing automatically in front of the TV or computer. As a final note, remember that most kids love to be involved in cooking and preparing food, given the chance. Get them kneading dough (satisfyingly messy) or dipping fresh fruit in melted 70% chocolate (just satisfying).

weblinks: www.ich.ucl.ac.uk – Institute of Child Health

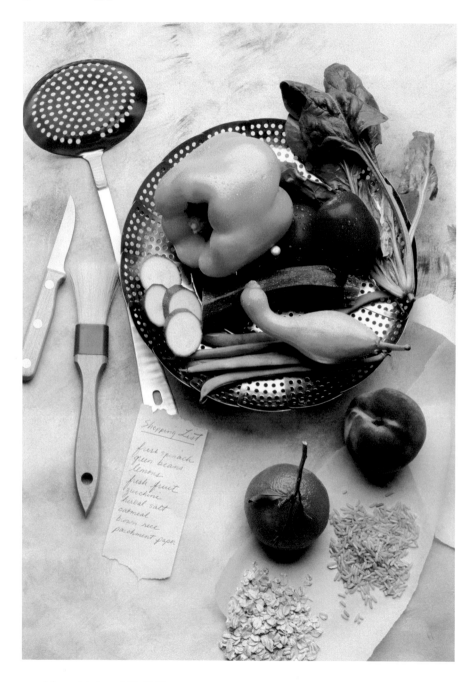

The GI+GL diet and older people

Eating the GI/GL way is suitable for anybody, no matter what their age, though there may be some special considerations. As people get older their metabolic rate decreases, so either exercise needs to be increased or calorie intake reduced appropriately. It is important that you try not to become unduly sedentary as you get older, and equally important that you don't put excess weight on. As you age, your sense of taste can become less acute, so you may add more salt to food to compensate, almost without realising it. Double-check your salt intake; high blood pressure is bad for anyone, and becomes an increasing health risk as you get older.

Cutting down on high-fat foods and eating more fibre will not only help to stop you becoming overweight, but will also protect you against some of the diseases that become more common with age. The risk of heart disease, for instance, increases dramatically once you reach middle age, so it makes sense to do what you can to mitigate that, and do it as soon as possible. If you are over forty and need to lose 5kg or more, talk to your doctor.

The GI+GL diet appeals to many older people because it's a return to healthier, 'old-fashioned' ways of eating. Those who have retired from work may have more time to cook meals from scratch using fresh ingredients, which is the ideal way to eat on the GI+GL diet.

want to know more?

▶ For more sensible and practical advice on your diet, you can contact a registered dietitian through the British Dietetics Association (0121 200 8080; www.bda.uk.com)
▶ The British Nutrition Foundation, a charity, also has advice on contacting registered dietitians or nutritionists (tel. 020 7404 6504; www.nutrition.org.uk)
▶ You can get your vitamin and mineral levels analysed and imbalances diagnosed for a fee by the following organisations: Biolab Medical Unit (UK) (tel 020 7636 5959; www.biolab.co.uk/tests) or The Natural Healthcare Centre (tel. 01283 516444; www.natural-healthcare-centre.co.uk).
▶ For advice on your child's weight, contact the Institute of Child Health (020 7242 9789, www.ich.ucl.ac.uk).
▶ See page 190 for a list of books about nutrition.

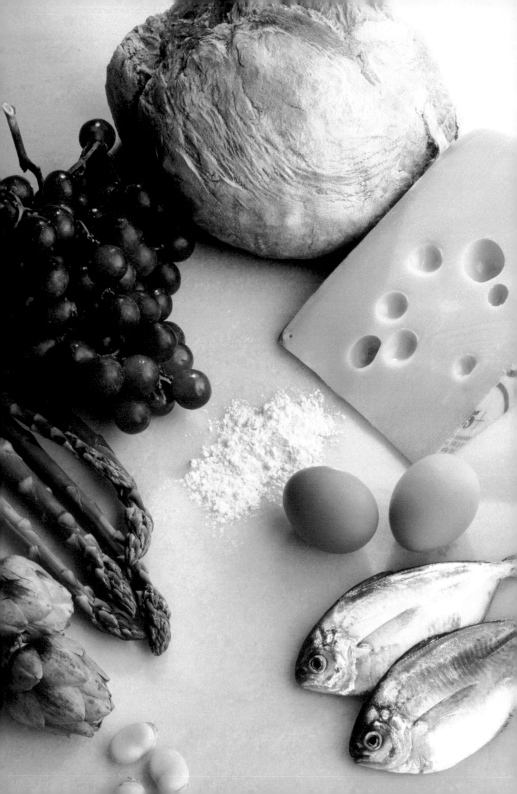

6 A diet for life

You've reached your target weight and the chocolate chip cookies are beckoning. Stop and consider before you give in. If you regain the excess weight and have to diet again, you risk confusing your metabolism so that it slows down. Then it would become harder to keep your weight stable in future. On the other hand, if you follow low GI/GL rules for life, you will be able to afford a few of those occasional treats *without* expanding your waistline.

A diet for life

You reached your target weight – congratulations! Now for staying there: and with the GI+GL diet, that doesn't have to be too much of a problem. Welcome to Part 2 of your diet.

You should have developed a taste for high-fibre loaves by now.

Stay healthy

Your health will already have improved significantly and it would be a shame not to build on that. The GI+GL diet isn't a 'Diet' as such, with a capital D, devoted only to weight loss; it's a healthy way of life and a general lifestyle change. What's so good about it is that it is easily sustainable without denying yourself in day-to-day life.

No patterns from the past

One word of warning. You may have managed to reach your target weight before on other diets and had the experience of seeing all the weight you had lost pile back on. Most successful dieters have. But the GI+GL is long term – not the same as those other diets – and, if you are careful and stick to the basic principles, regaining weight shouldn't be a problem. Don't adopt a mindset where you almost expect it to happen.

You will probably have reached your target in the past using a typical, restrictive diet – these ban you from eating certain food groups, or don't let you eat enough. Their only real aim is the weight loss itself; they don't attempt to alter the pattern of eating that put the weight on in the first place. As a result you don't make any permanent changes; the way you

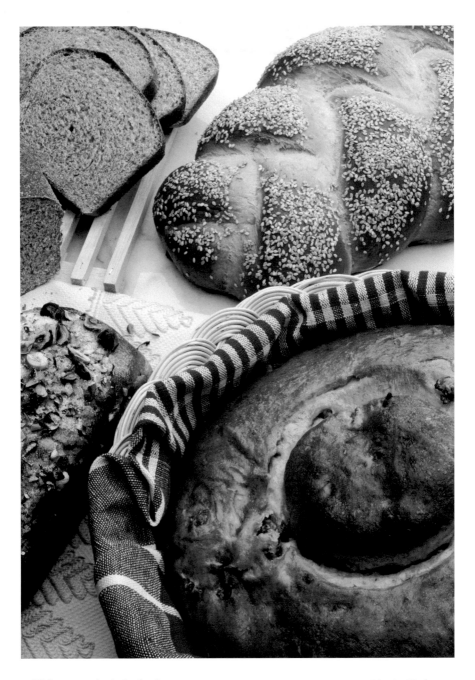

Opposite: The white rice in sushi has a high GL value, but the fish filling and nori wrapping help to lower the rating overall.

ate before is still there, lurking in the wings and ready to jump back on to centre stage when you stop dieting. Say you liked your carbs, but were on a carb-free or low-carb diet and were successful on it. The minute you reached target your first thought would naturally be 'Now I can eat toast and pasta again'. If you see your diet as an endurance test, something to slog through, then you are going to be relieved when it's over. There is no better way of concentrating your mind on something than telling yourself that you're not allowed to think about it. It's the old 'don't think of a pink elephant' trick – when somebody says that to you, you can't think of anything else, even if you deliberately say to yourself that you're not, no way, going to think about pink elephants. So if a diet says no bread at all, and you manage to stick to that for a while despite the fact that you love your bread, you end up thinking about it frequently – and the minute you stop dieting bread is there, right at the forefront of your mind.

This works another way, too. If you've had the weight regain experience in the past, you may be expecting it this time too. It's just what happens, right? Wrong. There's a theory, backed up by evidence from sport, that you really do get what you wish for, at least on one level. If football players think they'll miss a penalty, they do; if tennis players are convinced that their serves will hit the net, then they do. So if you're expecting weight gain you're inadvertently going to bring it about. It's a lot less likely – a lot – when you change to a GI/GL way of eating, but it's down to you, so stay positive. There are tools you can use to help you always make the right choices, ones that bring you to your long-term goal: staying at your target weight, and ensuring that you are healthier all round.

Practicalities

To keep your weight stable you have to bear in mind that energy in must equal energy out. Put in more energy (food) than your

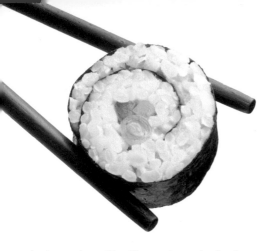

must know

Salad bars
Lots of supermarkets and restaurants have salad bars where you can make up your own combinations. Don't be tempted by any choices containing high-GL ingredients like pasta, or mixes which are drenched in dressing – and don't add dressing at the counter, either. You don't necessarily know what it contains.

body needs and it will store it, so the food you eat must balance the energy you expend. While you've been losing weight you've been taking in less energy than you've been using, and as a result your body has been using its fat reserves to make up the difference. You mustn't go on losing weight; that would undermine your efforts to be healthier. You have to balance everything, and stabilise your weight by taking in some extra energy.

This is absolutely not a licence to eat whatever you want regardless of quantity. Dieters who think this way will soon regain all the weight they've lost. Apart from anything else your resting metabolic rate (RMR) will have dropped while you were eating less. This isn't abnormal; it's the way our bodies – and the bodies of other animals – work. If food is scarce, the body adapts to manage with less energy. With a low GI+GL diet the reduction in RMR is less pronounced as your body is regulating the fuel it needs much better – you're eating to keep your blood sugar levels steady – but you still only need a slight increase in calories to balance your expenditure once you reach your target weight.

Part 2 of a GI+GL diet really isn't that different from Part 1. You still have to concentrate on eating healthily, and choosing mainly low- or no-GI/GL foods. Getting more exercise and general activity can help to boost your RMR and you should find it easier to keep fit because you'll have increased energy now you are at a healthy weight.

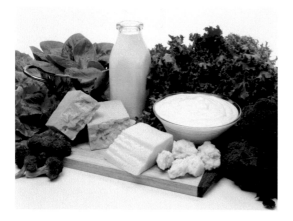

Dairy products and leafy green vegetables are rich in vitamins and minerals, especially calcium.

Energy in – food and drink

Continue to do all the things you were doing during your weight-loss period: not relying on manufactured food but eating as much freshly prepared food as you can; avoiding high-GI/GL carbs; eating regularly and not skipping meals; only eating healthy snacks... You'll probably find that some high-fat foods taste unpleasantly greasy and fatty now, and that you are repulsed by gigantic portion sizes. This makes it easier to maintain your new weight.

A way of increasing your calories carefully and gradually is to eat a few more medium GI or GL foods, or increase portion sizes a little. You could have 3 or 4 boiled new potatoes rather than 2 or 3, or a slightly larger portion of basmati rice, or a bigger helping of porridge at breakfast. You might have an extra slice of toast. You still need to be wary of the high, red-light GI and GL foods. This is also the stage where, if you stopped drinking alcohol completely in Part 1, you could reintroduce it. Gradually. The same is true of 70% dark chocolate.

The 'moderation, moderation, moderation' guideline still applies but you might care to add another slogan – 'quality, not quantity'. Buy seriously good chocolate and let it dissolve in your mouth; if you feel like a lamb chop or a steak, buy good-quality meat from an organic butcher; choose an excellent bottle of wine rather than the cheapest in the supermarket; go for a single malt rather than

must know

Water
Don't forget that dehydration, not just hunger, causes dipping energy levels. Aim to drink 8 glasses of water – around 1.5 litres – a day.

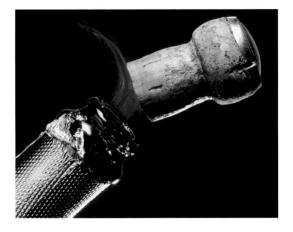

Holding out for nothing but the best is a good way to reduce the amount of alcohol you drink.

a 'this month's special offer' bottle of blended whisky. But always, always remember to drink alcohol with or immediately after food.

What to do if your weight goes up

If you find your weight creeping upwards, monitor it more closely: keep another food diary, which should help to isolate the problem. If your food intake seems to be going a bit haywire then you can use your diary to pinpoint the difficult times and problem foods. You might need to look at serving sizes, for example, but you won't realise that unless you keep tabs on what you're doing.

Make a note in your food diary about the mood you were in when you ate each meal or snack (especially the fattening ones). This could help you to pinpoint the causes. For example, you might find out that PMS is making things difficult, or that you are eating when you feel stressed. With PMS, accept that it is a temporary problem, lasting a few days at most, and don't beat yourself up. Your new diet, rich in omega-3 fatty acids, may even help.

must know

Successful losers
The National Weight Control Register in the US studies dieters who have each lost at least 14kg and kept it off for a year. It found that they all ate a low-fat diet, got plenty of exercise and weighed themselves regularly so they would spot the first signs of weight creeping back on.

weblinks: www.nwcr.ws – the site of the US National Weight Control Register

Eating when you are stressed can be more of a problem. It's perfectly normal, many people experience it, but understanding what is going on can help you deal with it. Stress eating is all to do with cortisol, a hormone which is part of the 'fight or flight' response, like adrenaline. It is there to 'mobilise' fuel – fat and glucose – and thus ensure peak performance when you really need it, but one of the side effects is that it increases your appetite. It also increases insulin levels. Levels of cortisol are higher among dieters anyway and one theory is that this is because dieting is stressful in itself. This is yet another reason why the GI+GL diet, which is more of a lifestyle change for slow and steady, gradual weight loss, with everything as unstressed as possible, is successful.

One way of dealing with increased cortisol is exercise. Go for a bit of flight – marching around the garden, running upstairs, going round the block to the post office – rather than reaching for the biscuits. There's a reason why you often feel the need to get out of the office after a stressful meeting, so act on it. Exercise actually releases chemicals that counteract stress and anxiety, calming you down. Not only are you less likely to chomp on chocolate, you're also less likely to take a bite out of someone close to you.

Energy out – exercise
One difference between people who manage to maintain their new weight and those who don't stands out clearly: exercise. Not necessarily team sports or spending hours in the gym, but a definite increase in physical activity.

By now you should be quite happy taking the more active option when there's a choice – climbing stairs rather than using a lift, walking rather than riding up escalators, or walking rather than taking the car. Keep an exercise diary, like your food diary

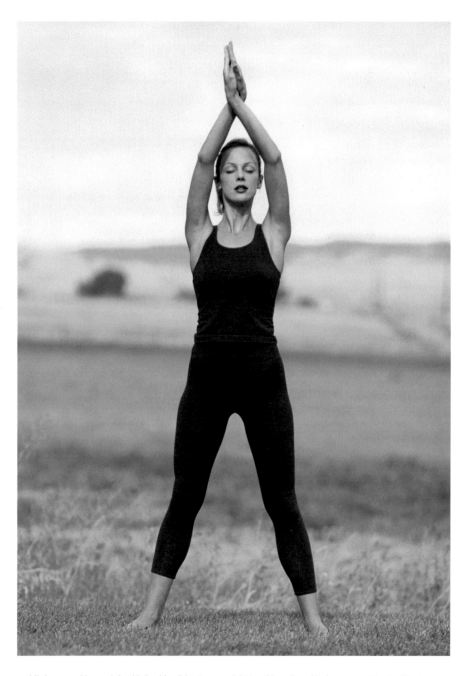

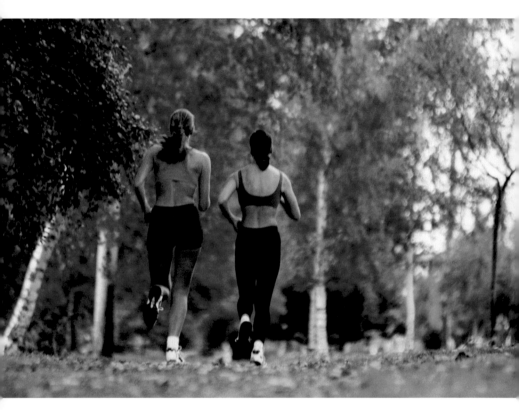

If you run, make sure you wear shoes that are specially designed for running, not just normal trainers.

(or combine the two), and record your activity level. If you couldn't take any exercise one day – perhaps it was pouring with rain or the dog was ill – record that fact and add the reason why as well. It's another tool you can use to help you keep your weight stable.

Even though this is the new, target-weight you, contemplating more exercise might still be distasteful... the answer to this is to get creative. Think about more unusual possibilities; you may find slightly off-the-wall suggestions more appealing than things that remind you of your schooldays. But do be sensible – there are some truly bizarre sports out there (bog snorkelling isn't for everyone) and some of the wilder adventure sports seem designed to kill you. How about learning to use a climbing wall, though? If you already do yoga, how about investigating astanga yoga, which is more energetic? Don't forget that dance counts as exercise, and there are often many alternative classes to choose from – jazz dance and salsa can use a lot of energy, but anything that gets you moving your body is good.

Then there's walking: move it up a gear from popping to the shops and walk quickly rather than dawdling. If you live in a city, start by really exploring it on foot. Play at being a tourist in your home town; tourist information offices may have leaflets with walking routes which would take you places you'd not normally visit and it can be surprising what's around the corner. Most cities in the UK are close to countryside, so make the most of it and go walking: marching up and down hills uses more energy than walking on the flat. If you already live in the country, then be a tourist there. Get some decent boots and explore your locality thoroughly. If you can't interest your family and friends in joining you, then go elsewhere: there are branches of the Ramblers' Association all over the country and they're usually friendly and non-competitive.

If the weather isn't conducive to walking, especially in winter, think about getting an exercise bike. Half an hour walking is the same as twenty minutes on such a bike. Yes, you can spend a lot of money but you don't have to; there are cheaper models, and it's possible to find good second-hand models by checking the small ads in local shops or newspapers. Make sure it's got – or can have – the right seat height for you and adjustable tension, and set it up somewhere by a radio or TV. It's surprising how quickly the time can pass once you're absorbed in an interesting programme, and it's also a good measure of time: you don't need to check every five minutes if you know you can stop when the programme ends.

must know

Calories burned by exercise
This depends on several factors, like body weight and how strenuously you exercise, but as a rule of thumb a 70kg person will burn 420 kcal an hour cycling, 530kcal jogging and 540kcal swimming.

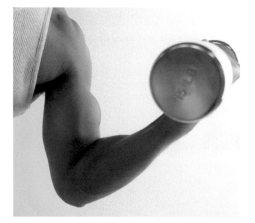

When using weights, it's better to do fewer repetitions at maximum effort than more with lighter weights.

Resistance exercise is vital for building muscle mass. Here you push against something – like your own body weight, stretch bands or free weights. You don't have to go to the gym; free weights are easily obtainable and can be used at home, as can bands. It's a good idea to go to a gym or exercise class to learn correct techniques before working with weights because you risk injury if you don't align your joints correctly. Push-ups are a form of resistance exercise where you push against your own body weight. Some types of aerobic exercise offer a measure of resistance – cycling, for instance, where your legs have to push the pedals.

Water provides more resistance than air, and working out in water is less likely to damage your joints. If you have weak joints, arthritis or are recovering from injury, it can be safer and just as effective as exercise out of water. It doesn't have to mean swimming up and down in lanes. Try aqua jogging, which burns twice as many calories as breaststroke, and doesn't have the injury potential of jogging on land. All you need is a buoyancy jogging vest (some pools hire these out) and a pool deep enough for your feet not to touch the bottom. Use the same movements as you would when running on land but flex and point your feet as you 'jog'. This helps your stability as well as strengthening the muscles at the front and back of your legs. You might get some odd looks at first, but ignore them (athletes with minor injuries often use this method of keeping fit). Don't forget to warm up before you begin – swim a couple of lanes without the vest on, then put it on and walk about in shallower water to get a feel for it. Always wind down afterwards with some gentle stretches.

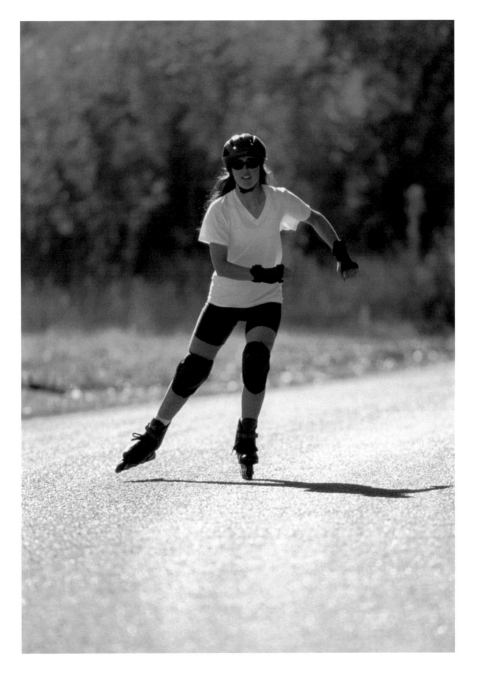

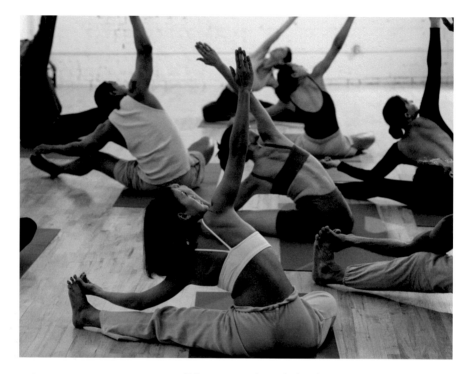

Joining a class can help to keep you motivated.

When you make a choice that suits you, motivation won't be a problem. You'll find yourself looking forward to your next climbing wall session – maybe to taking it a bit further with a weekend trip practising on the real thing – or to your next aquarobics class. There will be times when it's hard, when it's tedious to go to the pool on a cold day, when it's too windy to walk comfortably or when you're having a work crisis. That's just part of life, so don't be too hard on yourself; go back to the pool when it's a little warmer or buy a woolly hat...

The important thing is not to have unrealistic expectations because if you do, you are setting yourself up to fail. Attending a regular Pilates class if your nearest one involves an hour's journey counts as unrealistic; falling by the wayside would be almost inevitable in those circumstances. If you're an 'owl', at your liveliest at night, then expecting an early-morning running routine to last is unrealistic, too. Chop and change and find something that does fit into your lifestyle, and don't just restrict yourself to one activity. Experts recommend that you do at least three sessions of aerobic exercise a week, to give your heart and lungs a work-out, plus some kind of flexibility system like yoga, Pilates or weight training, to tone your muscles. There's bound to be something out there that suits you (but possibly not bog snorkelling).

Imagine...

A year from now. You'll be healthier, fitter; you'll feel fantastic and have much more energy. You'll have a much better chance of not developing heart disease, type 2 diabetes, some forms of cancer. And you'll have an understanding of the way your body works that will stand you in good stead for the rest of your life.

want to know more?

▶ See chapter 7 for low GI/GL recipes, chapter 8 for advice on eating out and chapter 9 for the GI/GL ratings of some common foods.

▶ *Collins Gem GI* and *Collins Gem GL* are handy pocket-size reference books that give comprehensive GI and GL ratings for foods and will help you to stick to your low GI/GL choices for life.

▶ For information on different types of exercises, see Joanna Hall's *The Exercise Bible*, or visit her website www.joannahall.com.

▶ *Collins Gem Pilates* and *Collins Gem Yoga* are useful introductions to these two types of exercise, which are great for flexibility and muscle strengthening.

▶ If you want to buy a pedometer to check how many steps you take in a day, visit www.pedometersuk.co.uk.

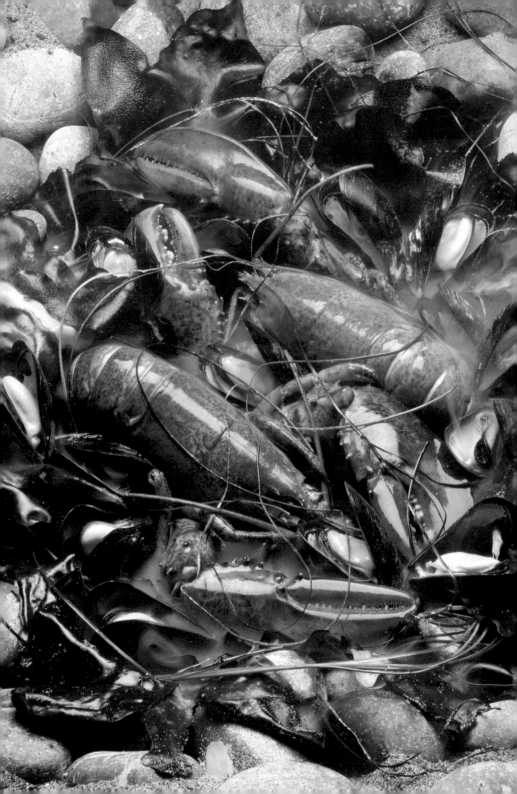

7 Low GI/GL recipes

All recipes serve four. Low GI/GL dieting is essentially healthy eating, so there is no need for the dieter to eat differently from anyone else. Just watch that you don't add high-calorie, high-GI/GL extras, such as crusty bread with soup, baked potatoes with fish or chicken, or sticky white rice with curry.

Italian chickpea, tomato and vegetable soup

A filling and nutritious lunch or supper dish.

Ingredients:

175g chickpeas, soaked
overnight

1 tsp olive oil

1 medium onion, sliced
into rings

1 clove of garlic, finely
chopped

1 small (230g) tin
chopped tomatoes

1 tsp mixed dried herbs

500g courgettes, sliced
into rings

125g other vegetables:
French beans, shelled
broad beans or peas

1 tbsp chopped parsley

salt and black pepper

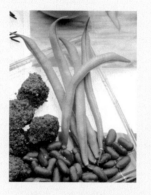

Some dried herb mixtures are more successful than others. Old favourites are often the best: 'herbes de Provence' are useful if you can get them, but classic 'mixed herbs' and 'Italian herbs' are equally good. Store them out of direct sunlight.

Drain the chickpeas and simmer them in fresh water until soft (at least 30 minutes). Skim off any froth that rises to the surface, then drain them over a bowl and reserve the cooking liquid.

Put the oil in a heavy saucepan over a high heat. Add the onion and garlic and cook until the onion begins to colour and soften. Reduce the heat, add the tomatoes and stir together for a minute or two. Then add the drained chickpeas, dried herbs, courgettes and enough of the cooking liquid from the chickpeas to cover – make the quantity up with water if necessary. Simmer, covered, for 5 minutes.

Now for the other vegetables. The best ones to choose are French beans or small broad beans (if the latter are large, they should be boiled briefly and skinned) or peas. Add these, together with the parsley, and cook for a further 5 minutes. Check the softness of the vegetables and the chickpeas – they should retain some bite – and season with a little salt and black pepper. Scatter with chopped parsley and serve.

Lentil and mushroom soup

Lentils are a good source of protein, without the fat found in red meat. Puy lentils would also work in this dish.

Ingredients:

150g green lentils

1 litre vegetable stock or
   water

1 medium onion,
   chopped

225g mushrooms, sliced

1 clove of garlic, chopped

1 tsp dried mixed herbs

a bay leaf

2 tsps tomato purée

150ml skimmed milk

salt and black pepper

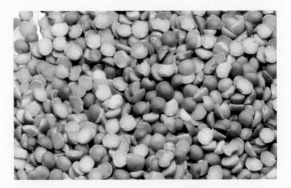

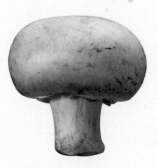

Rinse the lentils and check them for any small stones, just in case. They shouldn't need soaking in advance.

Heat the stock or water in a heavy saucepan; add the onion and let it cook a little. Add the mushrooms and continue cooking for another 2–3 minutes. Now add the lentils, garlic, dried herbs and bay leaf, and the tomato purée. Bring to the boil, then reduce the heat and cover the pan. Simmer until the lentils are soft – about 20 minutes.

Allow the soup to cool slightly and remove the bay leaf. Blend the soup in two halves, making one smoother than the other to vary the texture. Stir them together, add the milk and season with salt and black pepper. Reheat the soup gently – don't let it boil – and serve.

Haricot bean and parsley soup

A warming winter soup that can also be made with a mixture of different beans – try kidney, pinto or blackeyed beans.

Ingredients:

250g dried haricot beans, soaked
   overnight
2 tsps olive oil
3 sticks of celery, chopped
1 large onion, chopped
2 fat cloves of garlic, chopped
½ tsp paprika
water or vegetable stock
4 large handfuls of fresh parsley
black pepper

> **tip**
>
> Make your own stock. This doesn't have to
> involve simmering pans bubbling away for ages:
> just chop up an onion, a carrot and a small
> stick of celery. Put them in a pan, add some
> fresh parsley, a sprig of thyme and a bay leaf;
> cover everything with water. Simmer for 40
> minutes, then strain for a good vegetable stock.

Drain the haricots. Put them in a pan, cover with plenty of water, bring to the boil and boil for 10 minutes. Then reduce the heat, cover them and simmer for 20 minutes or until they're just soft. Check before that – if they're really fresh, they'll take less time. Drain, discarding the cooking water, and set them to one side.

Heat the oil in a large pan and cook the celery, onion and garlic until they soften. Then add the beans and the paprika, and stir everything together. Add enough water or vegetable stock to cover the beans and cook over a medium heat for 30 minutes.

Blend the soup in several batches, adding handfuls of fresh parsley to the blender with each one. Put everything back in the pan, add black pepper and check for seasoning; you don't want to dominate the fresh taste of the parsley. Reheat gently, and serve.

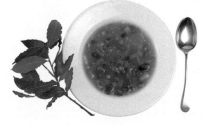

Aduki soup

Aduki beans are full of nutrients and have low GI/GL values and calorie counts. They're especially good for detoxing the system.

Ingredients:
125g dried aduki beans
2 tsps olive oil
1 red onion, chopped
1 carrot, chopped
2 cloves of garlic, chopped
4 tomatoes, chopped
1 tsp mixed dried herbs
water or vegetable stock
salt and black pepper

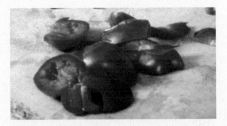

If you skin and deseed the tomatoes, you could keep some of the soup unblended (floating tomato skin looks messy and can get stuck in teeth). Score two lines around the tomato as though you were going to cut it in quarters, but just slitting the skin; the lines should cross at the base. Put them in a bowl and cover them with boiling water. Leave for a couple of minutes and then lift them out of the water, one by one, with a slotted spoon. You should be able to pull the skin from each 'quarter' easily, starting either where the lines meet or at the top.

Soak the aduki beans for three hours, then drain them and put them in a pan with fresh water. Bring to the boil; boil for 15 minutes, then lower the heat and simmer them for 15 minutes more. Test them – they should have softened nicely but retain a little bite; if they are a bit old they might need longer. Drain and discard the cooking water.

Warm the olive oil in a heavy saucepan, add the onion and carrot and cook until softened. Then add the beans, garlic, tomatoes and herbs, and enough water or stock to cover, and cook for 30 minutes. Season with salt and black pepper.

Remove from the heat and blend the soup in two batches, one more smoothly than the other. Mix the two batches together and serve.

Tuna and bean salad

Salads based on beans are great for you, but sometimes need a bit of a lift – this one has a good mixture of flavours and textures and would make an ideal light lunch.

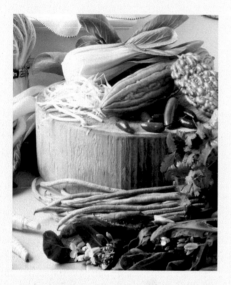

Drain the beans. Put them in a pan, cover them with plenty of water, bring them to the boil and boil for 10 minutes. Reduce the heat, cover the pan and simmer for 20 minutes or until they're soft. Drain them and leave to cool.

Drain and rinse the tuna and flake it in with the beans. Add the tomatoes, onion and black olives. Drizzle in a teaspoonful of good olive oil and a squeeze of lemon juice or dash of wine vinegar; season with salt and black pepper. Mix thoroughly and serve on a bed of salad leaves.

Ingredients:
125g dried haricot beans, soaked overnight
1 large (200g) can of tuna in brine, drained
2 chopped tomatoes
medium red onion, finely chopped
20 stoneless black olives, chopped
1 tsp olive oil
lemon juice or wine vinegar
salt and black pepper
mixed salad leaves

If your onion seems very strong when you first cut into it, soak it in a little salted water for five minutes or so. Squeeze it gently when you remove it, rinse and dry it and then slice it up.

Mexican fresh tomato salsa

This salsa – a traditional topping for tortillas – is great with grilled meat or fish, and makes a delicious snack if you scoop it up in cos lettuce leaves.

Ingredients:

4 large ripe tomatoes, deseeded and finely chopped

1 small red onion, finely chopped

20g fresh coriander, stems removed and then finely chopped

1 mild green chilli, very finely chopped (optional)

juice of 1 lime

black pepper

You might want to omit the chilli for children – or replace it with a stronger one for the more intrepid.

Don't use a blender to chop the ingredients as it will just pulp them; a food processor would be better, but best of all is a sharp knife or a half-moon-shaped chopper. Mix the chopped ingredients together in a bowl and squeeze the lime juice over everything. Add some black pepper, stir again and chill in the fridge for 20 minutes. It should not be kept for longer than four hours, so make it when you need it. If all the ingredients have been in the fridge you can dispense with the chilling.

Hummus

Once you've tried this, you'll never settle for ready-made, shop-bought hummus again...

Ingredients:

125g dried chickpeas, soaked
  overnight
juice of 2 lemons (or 1 if they are
  large and juicy)
2 tbsps tahini
2 cloves of garlic, finely chopped
1 tsp olive oil
paprika and parsley to garnish

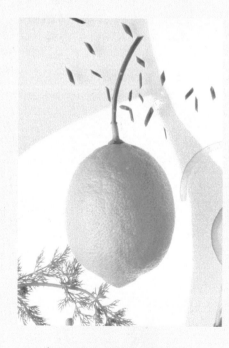

Drain the chickpeas and simmer in fresh water until they are soft – if they're fresh, this won't take very long (30 minutes or so). Skim off any froth that rises to the surface, then drain them over a bowl, reserving the cooking liquid. Put them in a blender or food processor with the lemon juice, tahini, garlic, olive oil and some of the cooking liquid. Don't add much of this liquid to start with – blend the mixture and see what the texture is like first before adding more; traditionally hummus is creamy but it's difficult to rescue if you add too much liquid.

When you're happy with the texture, put it into a bowl and sprinkle with a little paprika and chopped parsley. Hummus can be made in advance as it will keep, covered, in the fridge for a day or so (but don't put the paprika and parsley on until you are ready to serve).

Hummus is particularly good with raw vegetables to dip in it, especially spring onions, strips of carrot and cucumber, celery sticks, radishes and rings of fennel. A little wholemeal pitta could be used as well.

Horiatiki salata

This is the typical Greek summer salad. It's good with grilled or roast chicken fillets, grilled fish or lamb kebabs – or on its own.

Ingredients:

4 large ripe tomatoes, quartered
and seeds removed

1 medium onion, sliced into rings

1 green pepper, carefully deseeded
and sliced

½ a cucumber, peeled and thinly
sliced

sprigs of fresh thyme and oregano,
or a few basil leaves

black pepper

2 tsps olive oil

200g feta cheese

20 black olives

Put the tomatoes, onion, green pepper and cucumber together in a bowl. Remove the herb leaves from their woody stalks – or tear up the basil leaves – and scatter them over the salad, then add some black pepper to taste. Drizzle with the olive oil. Toss the salad gently together and transfer it to a serving dish or bowl.

Drain the feta and rinse it under cold running water. Pat it dry and crumble or slice it roughly over the salad. Scatter the olives on top and serve immediately – on a bed of cos lettuce, if you like.

Another traditional Greek salad which is ideal for the GI+GL diet is *fasolia salata*. You need 225g dried cannellini beans, soaked overnight and cooked, a chopped medium onion, 3 tbsps of chopped fresh parsley, salt and black pepper. Mix these together and dress them with a little olive oil and lemon juice. Garnish the salad with olives and hard-boiled eggs cut into quarters – and fresh oregano, if you can get it.

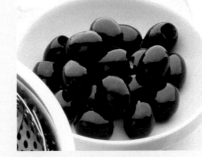

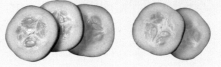

Tabbouleh

This Mediterranean salad used to be made with loads of cracked wheat, but fashions changed, giving it a much lower GI/GL rating.

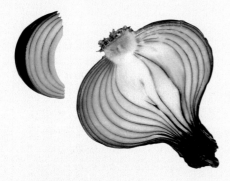

Ingredients:

80g cracked wheat

warm water or vegetable stock

juice from 1 lemon

black pepper

2 big bunches of flat-leaved
    parsley – you need about 200g
    without the stems

a large handful of fresh mint

1 small red onion, chopped

4 ripe tomatoes, chopped

2 tsps olive oil

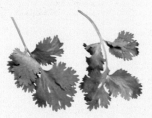

Cracked wheat, also called bulgur wheat, burghul or pourgouri, has already been partly cooked, so you only need to soak it in water or stock. Tabbouleh is lovely with plain grilled food or kebabs.

Half an hour before serving soak the cracked wheat in enough warm water or vegetable stock to cover it well. After about 15 minutes, test it – it should be soft. Drain and squeeze it dry. Put it in a bowl with the lemon juice and a little black pepper, stir it and leave it to soak up the juice.

Meanwhile, chop the parsley and mint finely – if you use a food processor to do this make sure you don't reduce them to a paste. Put the chopped herbs in a large serving bowl with the chopped onion and tomatoes, add the cracked wheat and the olive oil, and stir everything together thoroughly. The tabbouleh should be mostly green and red, with pale flecks of wheat. Serve immediately.

Salade Niçoise

There are lots of versions of this traditional salad (one even includes beetroot) but this goes back to the original.

Ingredients:

1 clove of garlic
8 medium tomatoes, quartered
1 cucumber, sliced
1 green pepper, thoroughly deseeded and sliced
8–10 spring onions, finely sliced
1 tsp oil
a squeeze of lemon juice
1 small tin of anchovies (50g)
250g tin of tuna in brine, rinsed and flaked
20 stoneless black olives
2 hard-boiled eggs, shelled and sliced lengthways
black pepper

Cut the garlic in half and rub the cut surfaces over the inside of the serving bowl, which should be wide rather than deep. Discard the garlic halves.

Put the tomatoes, cucumber, green pepper and spring onions in the bowl. Drizzle over the oil and a squeeze of lemon juice, and mix everything together. Now drain the anchovies, rinse off the oil and pat them dry on kitchen paper; arrange them decoratively on the salad. Scatter the flaked tuna over the top as well, and arrange the olives and hard-boiled eggs. Season with black pepper; the anchovies provide enough salt. Serve immediately.

If you like, you can serve this on a bed of lettuce – cos is best. You shouldn't feel the need for anything else with it, but traditional French sourdough bread – pain de campagne – is excellent.

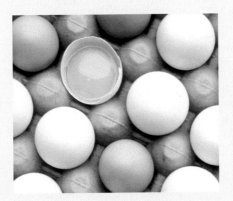

You can substitute fresh tuna for tinned. Lightly braise steaks for a few minutes on each side, so they are still pink in the middle.

Roast chicken breast fillets

These taste good hot or cold, can be used as a basis for all sorts of salads and could be part of a packed lunch.

Ingredients:

2 tsps olive oil

4 skinless chicken
    breast fillets

1 tsp mixed dried herbs

black pepper

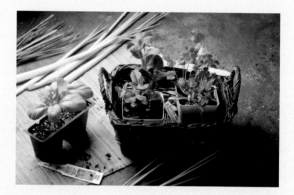

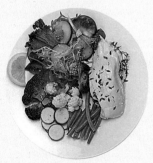

Heat the oven to 200°C /gas mark 6. Put the olive oil in an ovenproof dish big enough to hold all four fillets and pop it in the oven briefly. Rinse the fillets under running water and pat dry with kitchen paper, then remove the dish from the oven and roll the fillets over in the warm oil. Scatter the dried mixed herbs and grind a little black pepper over them, too.

Return the dish to the oven and roast the fillets for 15 minutes – after about 10, check the fillets and flip them over if necessary, then flip them back a couple of minutes later so the tops brown nicely. Serve hot or cold.

Lemon garlic chicken

A very lemony dish – and remember that lemon can help reduce the overall GI levels of a meal.

Ingredients:

2 tsps olive oil

4 skinless chicken breasts

1 medium red onion, chopped

2 large sprigs of fresh thyme

4 cloves of garlic, halved

2 organic unwaxed lemons

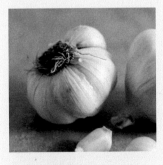

Always buy organic lemons, limes and oranges if you can: pesticides can easily penetrate the rind of citrus fruit. You'll need to keep them in the fridge.

Preheat the oven to 200°C /gas mark 6. Put the oil into a large ovenproof dish and pop it in the oven briefly to warm up. Meanwhile, rinse the chicken pieces and pat them dry. Remove the dish from the oven and roll the chicken pieces over in it, coating them with the warm oil. Add the chopped onion and strip the leaves from the stems of thyme; scatter the leaves over the chicken fillets and tuck the garlic halves around them.

Cut the lemons in half and squeeze them by hand over the chicken, then cut each lemon portion in half and put them in the dish too; don't worry about the pips. Return the dish to the oven and bake the chicken for 15 minutes, then take it out and turn the chicken over. There will be quite a lot of liquid in the dish. After another 5 minutes, turn the pieces back. By now the liquid should almost all have evaporated and you want the chicken pieces to brown a little. Bake for another 5 minutes and test that the chicken is cooked.

Serve, resisting the urge to scrape caramelised juice off the sides of the dish. Leave the garlic halves and lemon pips in the ovenproof dish; give each person a couple of lemon portions with their chicken, and some onion. Scrape the soft pulp out of the lemons and eat it with the chicken. Serve with a crisp green salad (no salad dressing is necessary).

Masoor dhal with courgettes and tomatoes

This tasty Indian dish comes highly recommended...

Ingredients:

250g red lentils

1 onion, chopped

water or vegetable stock

2 tsp rapeseed oil

1 tsp black mustard seeds

2 large courgettes, chopped

2cm cube of fresh ginger, chopped

2 chopped cloves of garlic

1 tsp turmeric

1 tsp garam masala

3 large tomatoes, skinned, deseeded and chopped

juice of 1 lemon

50ml water

salt and black pepper

fresh coriander for garnish

Try this relish if you like raw onion. Thinly slice an onion into rings and mix them with lemon juice, a little black pepper and salt. Leave to stand for an hour, transfer the onion to a serving dish and sprinkle with paprika.

Rinse the lentils and put them in a pan with a small handful of the chopped onion. Cover well with water or vegetable stock and bring to the boil. Remove the froth as it rises (the onion makes this a little awkward but it doesn't matter if some ends up in the sink with the froth). Stir the lentils occasionally as they have a tendency to clump together. Reduce the heat and simmer for 20 minutes.

Meanwhile heat the oil in a large pan which has a lid. Add the mustard seeds, cover the pan and cook them until they start popping against the lid. Then add the rest of the onion, the courgette, ginger and garlic and fry gently, stirring, for about 5 minutes – they should brown but not burn. Add the turmeric and the garam masala and stir for a further minute, then add the tomatoes, lemon juice, about 50 ml water and some salt and pepper. Simmer for another couple of minutes, stirring from time to time.

Drain the lentils thoroughly and add them to the pan with the vegetables and the spices. Stir them together well and cook until the liquid has evaporated – probably a further 3 minutes or so.

Garnish with coriander leaves and serve with a raita, accompanied by chapatis (but without any of the ghee or oil which is sometimes used on them – see page 151) or a wholemeal pitta.

Cucumber raita is easy. Grate a cucumber, then squeeze out the excess liquid using your hands. Stir the now much drier grated cucumber into low-fat natural yoghurt and serve it as an accompaniment. If you like the taste, you could add some garlic too, or maybe some chopped raw onion. Raita is also delicious with kebabs and grilled chicken or fish.

Mild chicken and spinach curry

This curry is deliberately mild, so that the flavours of the chicken and the spinach come through.

Ingredients:

4 skinless chicken breast fillets

1 tsp rapeseed oil

1 large onion, chopped

2 cloves of garlic, finely chopped

4 medium tomatoes, chopped

1 tsp ground cumin

1 tsp ground coriander seeds

½ tsp cayenne pepper

black pepper

4 cardamoms (optional)

450g fresh spinach, any thick stalks removed, washed and roughly chopped

salt

60ml natural yoghurt

Cut the chicken into pieces roughly 2cm square. Heat the oil in a heavy pan and brown the chicken pieces. Once they have begun to colour remove them with a slotted spoon and set them aside. Add the onion and garlic to the pan and fry until they begin to soften, then add the tomatoes. Keep stirring so it doesn't burn; it will be quite dry but don't be tempted to add any more liquid.

When the tomatoes have begun to soften add the cumin, coriander, cayenne and a little black pepper. Stir a little more and then add the cardamoms, if using, and return the chicken to the pan. Then add the chopped spinach and a little salt.

Keep stirring until the spinach wilts and begins to give off liquid, then cover the pan and simmer the curry over a medium heat, stirring occasionally, for 30 minutes or until the chicken is tender. You may find that you need to raise the heat and uncover the pan to evaporate some of the liquid – this isn't a dry curry, but it shouldn't be drowned.

Remove the pan from the heat and, once it has stopped bubbling, carefully stir in the yoghurt – if the curry is still boiling the yoghurt will separate. If you can find them, remove the cardamoms; otherwise simply warn people – they're just surprisingly chewy. Serve immediately.

This curry is deliberately mild, so that the flavours of the chicken and the spinach come through. It's good served with basmati rice or chapatis and a fresh, leafy salad.

Cassoulet with cod

The French classic is usually made with sausage, but this fish version is much healthier.

Ingredients:

175g dried haricot beans, soaked
  overnight
2 tsps olive oil
2 leeks, chopped into rings
1 medium onion, chopped
2 cloves of garlic, chopped
500g cod loin
4 tomatoes, skinned, deseeded
  and chopped
a large sprig of fresh thyme
black pepper
a bay leaf
100ml dry white wine
50ml vegetable stock or water

Drain the beans. Put them in a pan, cover with plenty of water, bring to the boil and boil for 10 minutes. Reduce the heat, cover and simmer until they're tender – about 20–30 minutes, depending on the freshness of the beans. Drain them again, discarding the cooking water.

Preheat the oven to 180°C /gas mark 4, and put a casserole inside to warm up. Heat the oil in a pan over a medium heat and cook the leeks, onion and garlic for 5 minutes until they are soft. Meanwhile cut the cod loin into chunks about 2cm square, getting rid of any bones you might encounter (there shouldn't be many).

Put the leek and onion mixture into the casserole that's been warming in the oven. Add the beans, tomatoes and thyme; stir well and then add the cod and stir again, more gently. Season with black pepper, pop in the bay leaf and pour the wine and water or stock over.

Cover the casserole and bake the cassoulet for 30 minutes. Check to see how it is doing at this point and cook a little longer if the fish seems to need it; it probably won't. Serve immediately, removing the bay leaf.

This is ideal served with lots of steamed mangetout or lightly cooked courgettes – it's also good with a green salad. It's substantial enough not to need rice or potatoes.

good, easy quick

Provençal chicken

A tasty French country casserole. Serve with a green salad and a little brown rice or a slice of wholemeal bread.

Ingredients:

4 skinless chicken breasts

12 small onions or shallots, whole but trimmed and peeled

2 tsps olive oil

1 red onion, sliced into rings

1 green pepper, sliced

2 cloves of garlic, chopped

1 large (400g) tin of chopped tomatoes

a pinch of mixed dried herbs

100ml stock or water

salt and black pepper

20 stoneless black olives

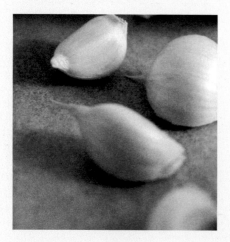

Brown the chicken pieces and the small onions, using a teaspoon of the oil in a heavy saucepan or ovenproof casserole over a high heat. Once they are slightly coloured, remove them and put to one side. Reduce the heat and put another teaspoon of oil in the pan. Then add the sliced onion, green pepper and garlic; soften these for 5 minutes. Return the chicken and small onions to the pan; add the tomatoes, herbs and stock. Taste and season with salt and black pepper.

Cover the pan and cook gently until done – about 40–45 minutes on top of the oven, or about 55 minutes inside the oven at 180°C/gas mark 4. Halfway through, turn the chicken over and stir the pan gently – the liquid should be relatively low; this isn't a stew, but nor should there be any danger of the chicken sticking. If you do have a lot of cooking liquid, then leave the lid off the pan for the rest of the cooking time; add some extra if it looks low.

About 10 minutes before the time is up, add the olives. Stir well, but gently, before serving.

Chilli beans

These baked beans are delicious and spicy, but be careful with your chilli powder – some varieties are stronger than others.

Ingredients:

200g dried haricot beans, soaked
   overnight
1 tsp olive oil
1 large onion, sliced and roughly
   chopped
1 large clove of garlic, chopped
½ tsp ground cumin
1 tsp dried mixed herbs
½ tsp chilli powder (or to taste)
1 large (400g) tin of chopped
   tomatoes
½ tsp sugar

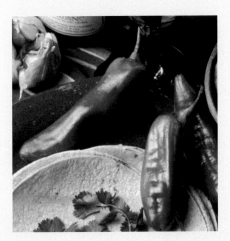

Drain the beans. Put them in a pan, cover with plenty of water, bring them to the boil and boil for 10 minutes. Then reduce the heat, cover the pan and simmer for 20 minutes or until they're soft. Check before that – the fresher they are, the less time they'll take. Drain them over a bowl to retain the cooking liquid.

Heat the oil in a heavy pan. Add the onion and cook for 2–3 minutes, then add the garlic and cook for another couple of minutes, but don't let the garlic brown. Stir in the cooked beans, the ground cumin, mixed herbs and chilli powder. Cook, stirring, for another 2–3 minutes.

Add the tomatoes, sugar and enough of the cooking liquid to just cover the beans. Cover the pan and cook for 40–45 minutes (test it for chilli hotness after about 10 minutes). Check the level of the liquid every so often, stirring to prevent the beans from sticking. You don't want to end up with a lot of juice – just keep it moist.

Serve with a crunchy green salad.

Oriental salmon

The oriental flavours of this dish go well with basmati rice, and possibly some steamed broccoli on the side.

Ingredients:

2 sticks of lemon grass, chopped into a few large pieces
4 salmon fillets or steaks
2 tbsps sherry or white vermouth
1 tbsp dark soy sauce
juice of 1 lemon
6 spring onions, sliced
1 clove of garlic
2cm cube of fresh ginger

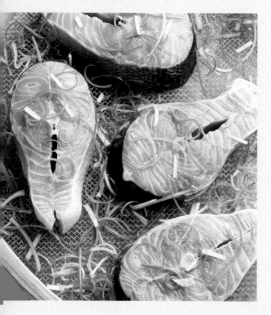

Preheat the oven to 200°C /gas mark 6. Put the sticks of lemon grass in an ovenproof dish and place the salmon on top. Pour the sherry or vermouth, soy sauce and lemon juice into the dish, and spoon it over the fish. Scatter the salmon with the spring onion, then finely grate the garlic and the ginger over it. Spoon the liquid over everything once more, and put the dish in the oven. Cook for 15 minutes. Halfway through check to make sure that some liquid still remains: if your lemon was juicy you should be fine, if it looks a little low, cover the dish with foil. Cook for a further 15 minutes and check that the salmon is cooked – this will depend on the thickness of the fillets.

Leave the lemon grass in the dish and put the salmon on warmed plates. Spoon a little liquid over each fillet before serving.

Salmon packets with herbs

Salmon can sometimes be dry – but not cooked like this. Serve with steamed vegetables, or cold with a mixed herb salad.

Ingredients:

4 salmon fillets, about 125g each

2 bay leaves

4 sprigs each of parsley and thyme

2 slices of onion

2 slivers of unwaxed lemon rind
    and a squeeze of juice

black pepper

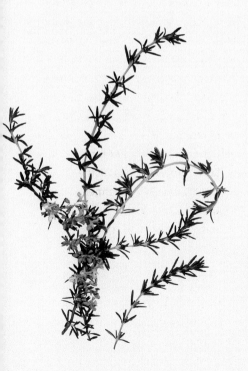

Preheat the oven to 200°C /gas mark 6. Have two squares of foil ready, each big enough to wrap two fillets up generously. Place two pieces of fish side by side on each square. Divide the bay leaves, sprigs of parsley and thyme, onion and lemon rind evenly between the two parcels, placing them on top of the salmon and tucking some between the fillets, which stops them sticking together. Squeeze a little lemon juice over, and season lightly with black pepper. Fold the foil up and around the fillets loosely, tucking the edges together to make sure no steam can escape.

Put the foil packets in an ovenproof dish and bake in the oven for 15 minutes.

Be careful opening the packets, as hot steam will escape; discard the wilting herbs and onion before serving.

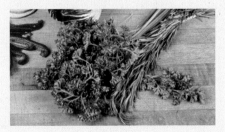

Spiced pears

Non-dieters might enjoy crème fraiche with this tasty dessert. Dieters should stick to a low-fat brand...

Ingredients:

100ml dry white wine

100ml water

a pinch of grated nutmeg

a small piece of cinnamon stick
   (about 2cm long)

grated rind of half an organic,
   unwaxed orange

4 ripe pears

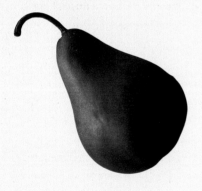

Put the wine, water, nutmeg, cinnamon and orange rind in a saucepan. Bring to the boil, cover and simmer for 5 minutes, checking every so often to make sure the liquid isn't boiling away completely.

Wash the pears, cut them in quarters and core them. Put them into the liquid and poach them, covered, for 20 minutes or until they are soft – this will depend on their variety and ripeness. Look at them during this time, and give them a gentle stir, to make sure all the quarters are cooking and that they're not sticking.

Have four plates ready. Once the pears are cooked remove them from the pan using a slotted spoon, arrange four quarters on each plate and let them cool a little. If there's quite a bit of liquid left, boil it up a bit more until it reduces – you should have about 2–3 tablespoons. Drizzle it over the pears and serve.

Atholl brose

A healthy version of this rich Scottish pudding. Even so, a little goes a long way.

Ingredients:

20g jumbo oats
10g flaked almonds
300g no-fat Greek yoghurt
1 tsp clear honey
1 tbsp whisky
a squeeze of lemon juice

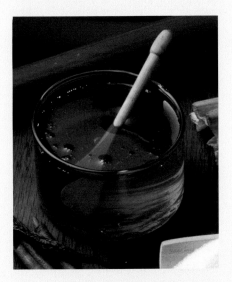

Put the oats and the flaked almonds in a dry baking tray under a hot grill – keep an eye on them, stirring them around to make sure they don't burn but colour evenly. When they are golden-brown and beginning to smell warm and toasted, remove the baking tray and pour them onto a plate to cool.

Mix the yoghurt, honey and whisky together carefully. Add almost all the toasted oats and almonds, reserving some to use as decoration. Squeeze in a little lemon juice and fold everything together thoroughly. Divide the mixture equally between four ramekin dishes, sprinkle with the reserved oats and almonds, and serve.

This is best served immediately. If necessary it can be kept for a couple of hours in the fridge, but don't add the decorative topping until just before serving.

Baked apple slices

Although it's just made from fruit, this dish is surprisingly rich so you don't need a lot.

Ingredients:

4 small dessert apples, quartered
   and cored but with skin left on
2 tsps raisins or sultanas
8 dried apricots, chopped
grated rind and juice of half an
   orange
½ tsp cinnamon
½ tsp brown sugar
low-fat crème fraîche

Preheat the oven to 180°C /gas mark 4. Line the insides of four ramekin dishes tightly with the apple quarters; the curve of the fruit and the curve of the dish will match well and leave you with a gap in the centre. Mix together the raisins, apricots, orange rind and cinnamon, and fill the centre gaps with this mixture. Drizzle the orange juice over everything and then sprinkle a little brown sugar on top of each ramekin, concentrating on the apple slices.

Bake them for 15 minutes. To serve, tip each pot gently onto the middle of a plate and accompany with a little low-fat crème fraîche.

The same filling can be used with whole cooking apples. Core the apples, put them on pieces of foil big enough to wrap them up and fill the core gap with the raisin, apricot, orange peel and cinnamon mix. Pour the juice on top of the filling, wrap the apples (sealing the foil) and bake them until they are soft to the touch. Be careful opening the foil as steam will escape.

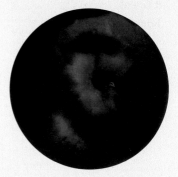

Strawberry yoghurt fool

Fruit fools are delicious, but high in calories – it's all that double cream and sugar. This is a healthier alternative.

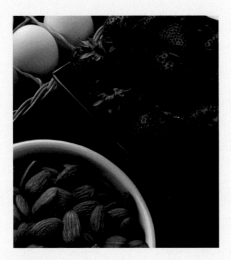

Ingredients:
200g very ripe strawberries, trimmed
300g no-fat Greek yoghurt
1 tsp clear honey
4 tsps flaked almonds
a few mint leaves for garnish

Reserve some of the strawberries for decoration and use a fork to mash the rest up in a bowl. Drain off some of the resulting liquid and keep it in the fridge.

Add the yoghurt to the pulped strawberries and fold it in, incorporating the fruit. Add the honey and mix that in well. Then spoon the mixture into four ramekin dishes, cover and chill for a couple of hours.

Just before you're ready to serve, toast the flaked almonds in a dry frying pan, stirring them to make sure they don't burn; they should be golden-brown in colour. Set them aside to cool. Put each ramekin on a plate and place some whole strawberries beside it; drizzle some of the reserved juice over them and garnish with a couple of mint leaves. Crumble the toasted almonds roughly and scatter them over the tops of the ramekins. Serve immediately. It's not as solid as a high-fat, high-GI fool, so don't be tempted to top it with fruit as it would just sink.

Nectarines with summer fruits

A delicious summery dessert, best made when soft fruits are locally in season.

Ingredients:

75g raspberries

1 tbsp Cointreau or Grand Marnier

2 ripe nectarines

40g blueberries

200g strawberries, trimmed and
   chopped

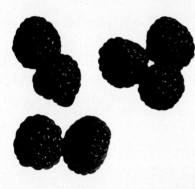

Squeeze the raspberries through a sieve into a bowl using a wooden spoon – at first you get very little purée coming through, but soon the seeds are almost the only thing left in the sieve. Scrape the last drops of purée off the underside of the sieve into the bowl, too; it doesn't look like a lot, but don't be tempted to add more. Mix the Cointreau or Grand Marnier into the pulped raspberries. Slice the nectarines into the purée and stir the slices gently to coat them in raspberry pink. Then add the blueberries and strawberries and mix everything together. Put into serving dishes and serve immediately if all the ingredients have been in the fridge; otherwise chill for a couple of hours.

Chapatis

A classic accompaniment for Indian meals, with much lower GI/GL values than naan bread or pilau rice.

Ingredients:
100g stoneground wholemeal flour
25ml water

Put the flour in a bowl and add the water little by little, mixing it with the flour until it sticks together and becomes kneadable – you probably won't use all the water. Knead the dough for 10 minutes until it is smooth, then cover it with a damp cloth and put it aside to rest for 30 minutes.

Put a big plate with a napkin spread over it to one side in a warm place – as you cook the chapatis, pile them up and fold the napkin over them so they stay warm while you cook the rest. You should also have more flour ready to use when you roll them out. Heat a heavy frying pan, without any oil in it, on top of the stove.

Knead the dough again and divide it equally into 8 pieces. Form these into small balls and keep the ones you aren't using under the damp cloth. Flour a surface big enough to roll them out and take out the first ball. Flatten it between your fingers, dusting it well with flour, and then roll it. You will need to turn it round a lot, turn it over frequently and keep the surface well dusted with flour if it is not to stick. You should be able to make a chapati about 12cm in diameter.

The pan should be hot by now. Pat the chapati to shake off excess flour, then lay it in the pan. When the upper side begins to bubble and develop whiter areas, look underneath – tiny brown spots should be beginning to appear on the underside. Flip it over, using tongs, and cook the other side.

If your pan is at the right temperature, the first side should take about 20–30 seconds, and the second side less than half that – if it's too hot the bread will burn before cooking; if it's not hot enough it will be leathery. You'll soon get a feel for it; all cookers or hobs – and pans – are different.

Put your first chapati on the napkin and fold the sides over it, covering it well. Cook the rest in the same way and serve as soon as the last one is done.

Seeded wholemeal bread

This is the quickest, easiest bread recipe and makes 2 x 450g (1 lb) loaves. Any yeast marked 'fast', 'quick' or 'easy' will do. If you use ordinary dried yeast, you'll need one tablespoon – follow the instructions on the packet for reconstituting it. Fresh yeast is almost impossible to find.

Ingredients:

2 tsps wheat grain

1 tsp linseeds

1 tsp pumpkin seeds

1 tsp sunflower seeds

650g stoneground wholemeal flour

2 tsps salt

1 tsp sugar

2 tsps 'easy bake' yeast

1 tbsp olive oil

400ml warm water (one part boiling to two parts cold gives the right temperature)

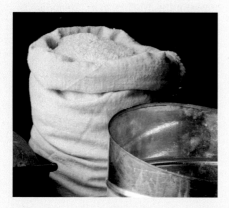

Grind the grain and seeds briefly in a coffee grinder or mortar and pestle (or put them in a strong, sealable plastic bag and use a rolling pin); some should stay whole. You can leave them all whole, but pumpkin and sunflower seeds are rather large.

Warm a big mixing bowl and at the same time put two 450g loaf tins in the oven to warm. In the bowl stir together the flour, salt, sugar, yeast and the ground seed mixture; add the oil and mix thoroughly. Now add the warm water and mix to a soft doughy consistency. Knead the dough for 10 minutes – you can use a floured surface but doing it in the bowl is fine and a lot less messy. You don't have to thump the dough; just knead it firmly, pushing it and turning it. You may find that you need to sprinkle on more flour if it becomes too sticky, but it should be nicely elastic, springing back when you prod it.

Oil the two warmed tins so the bread won't stick, and divide the dough

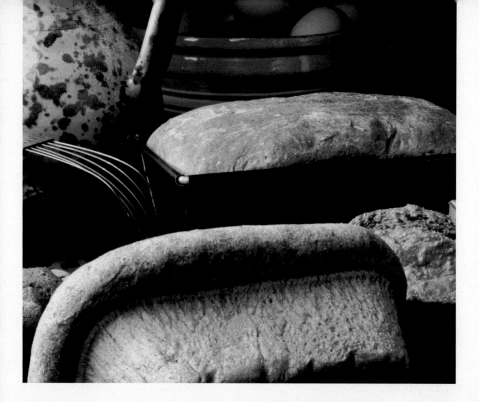

between them. Cover the tins loosely and leave them in a warm place so the dough can rise for about 30 minutes – it should almost double in size. Preheat the oven to 230°C/gas mark 8.

Spray the tops of the loaves with water and place the tins in the middle of the oven. Bake for 30–35 minutes, but check them after about 10... all ovens are different and you may need to protect your bread with a sheet of foil to prevent the loaves burning.

When they are cooked, remove the tins from the oven and turn them out after a couple of minutes – the loaves are ready when they sound hollow when you tap the underside. Cool them on a wire rack, and don't try and slice them neatly while they are still warm; it's impossible!

Bread made with 'quick' yeasts only needs one rising, but a second will make the loaf even better. After kneading, give your dough a first, 30-minute rise in the bowl, covered with a cloth, then knock it back and knead it again – but carefully this time, don't tear it. Divide it into the warmed tins and let it rise again for 30 minutes. Generally, the slower the rise, the better the bread.

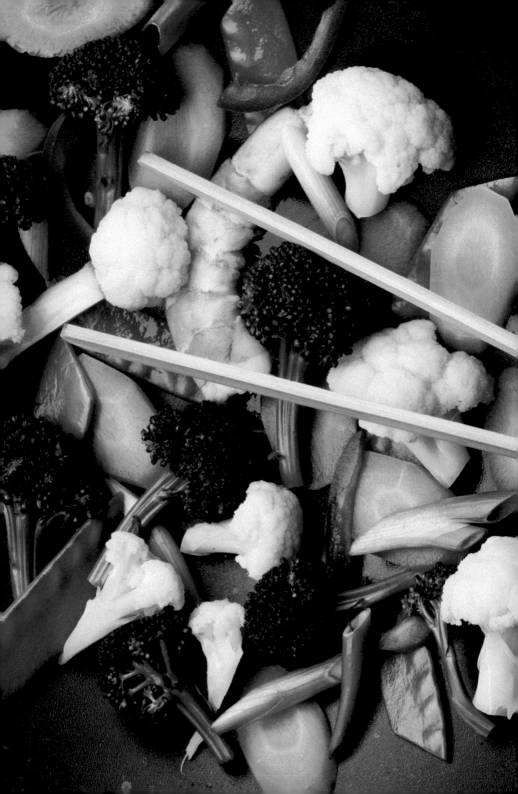

8 Eating out

There is a huge variety of places to eat, ranging from expensive restaurants to fast-food outlets, and covering cuisines from all over the world. Good GI/GL choices are almost always possible, but so are problem areas. In this chapter you'll find some guidelines. The cuisines are listed alphabetically, with fast food at the end – and then party food, where many of the same general principles apply.

Eating out

On many diets it's almost impossible to go out for a meal. That's not true of the GI+GL diet, once you understand the way it works, and providing you stick to its principles. But the best choices in restaurants are not always obvious, and some cuisines are more GI-friendly than others.

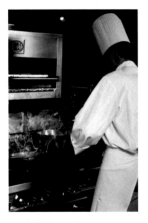

Remember that cooking methods can affect GI/GL values.

General rules

If you know you are going out in the evening, don't deliberately starve yourself during the day, which would mean you were ravenous by the time you sat down and opened the menu. If you have a quick, low-GI snack before you go out, it will take the edge off your appetite and make it easier for you to stick to your diet. Then:

▶ Drink some water before eating anything in the restaurant or café.

▶ Keep your choices clear and simple.

▶ Don't be shy about asking the waiter to explain what each dish contains.

▶ If you are offered bread, decline – unless it looks as though it might be low GI.

▶ Don't have chips; if they come with the dish you are ordering, ask if you can substitute something else, like a salad or an extra vegetable. The same applies to potatoes.

▶ Don't order all your courses at the start of your meal – that's a sure-fire way to choose a tempting pud.

▶ Eat slowly and really enjoy your food.

▶ Watch your alcohol intake. By all means, drink a couple of glasses of wine with the meal, but remember that you've just consumed 200 or so extra calories.

▶ Despite what you might have been told when you were little, it's fine to leave food on your plate if you are full.

British

Go for basic foods, simply cooked. Say yes to chicken, grilled lean meat and simple roast meat, but trim off any obvious fat – and no pork crackling, floury or fatty gravy, Yorkshire puddings or roast potatoes. Classic British fish dishes are a good choice: opt for Dover sole, grilled herrings or kippers, poached smoked haddock, local oysters or mussels. Try to operate the plate portion control rule, filling half your plate with vegetables.

Keep in mind the general rules and don't go anywhere near pies, pastries or traditional sticky puddings, with or without custard. If you crave a dessert, they may have baked apples or poached pears, which would be alright if eaten without cream, custard or ice cream. Also avoid the full English breakfast, any fish with batter or breadcrumbs, chips and fried food. Beer is out... see page 83 if you can't remember why.

Ask for extra vegetables instead of chips or potatoes.

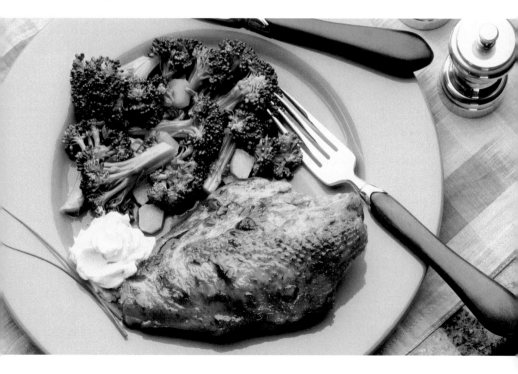

Chinese

Chinese food can be tricky; the rice is almost always high GI/GL, and noodles aren't any better. The other danger to watch out for is helping yourself to other people's high-GI/GL choices; Chinese restaurants are frequently sociable places and food tends to be shared. You can say yes to clear soups, stir-fried vegetables, chicken or beef (but without thick sauces), baked and grilled fish, and boiled cellophane noodles. You need to avoid rice, any noodles except those cellophane ones (and not those if they've been fried), sesame prawn toasts and dim sum, anything at all that is in a sweet and sour sauce, Peking duck with pancakes and – of course – toffee apples or bananas.

French

Stick to plain dishes like grilled steak or trout with almonds. Salade Niçoise is a good choice (but watch out for the potatoes included in some versions), as is cassoulet, a dish made from haricot beans and meat. When you think of French bread you tend to think of baguettes (no way) but the French actually eat a lot of good sourdough bread, usually called 'pain de campagne', which is worth looking out for as an alternative. Definite no-nos include garlic bread, potatoes and chips, cream sauces, bread – including croissants and those baguettes – quiches and tarts, crêpes and any chocolatey and creamy desserts like profiteroles.

Greek and Middle Eastern

There are some great low-GI/GL choices in these restaurants, but many dishes will involve a lot of oil.

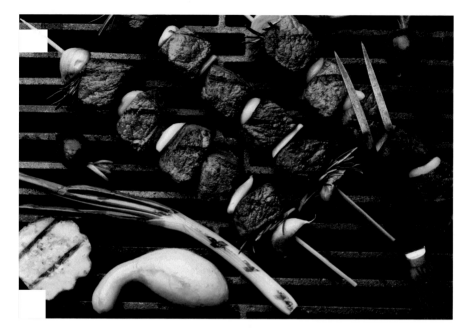

Grilled food is a safer bet, whether it's meat, fish or in the form of kebabs. In addition to grilled food, Middle Eastern restaurants often use beans, lentils and nuts, and side salads are usually available. Greek salad is a good choice, and hummus, taramasalata and tsatsiki are fine with raw vegetables to dip in them. Olives are ideal and many mezze – little appetisers – are good too, if you resist the impulse to eat a lot of pitta bread with them. Avoid dolmades (rice-stuffed vine leaves) and moussaka, which has a potato topping. Squid is often fried in batter, and meatballs and sausages are out too. In Middle-Eastern restaurants cous-cous should be declined, as should tabbouleh – make your own version of this refreshing salad at home instead (see page 134). Sticky Greek and Middle-Eastern puddings are out too, and 'Turkish' coffee is usually very sweet.

Grilled or barbecued kebabs with lots of vegetables is a good choice at home or in a restaurant.

weblinks: www.weightlossresources.co.uk/diet/eating_out

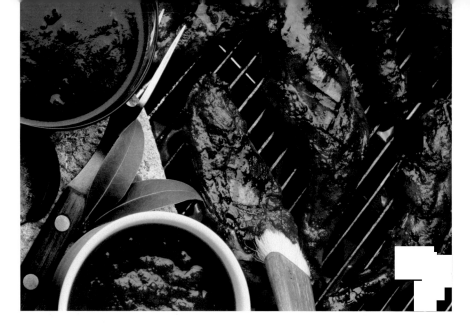

Tandoori is one of the best choices in an Indian restaurant.

Indian

There are many possible choices on the menu of most Indian restaurants. Rice is usually plain, boiled basmati, so go for that and don't be tempted by any variations, biryanis or pilaus. Tandoori dishes are an excellent option, though you should avoid any breads or popadoms. The latter are usually deep-fried, though some brands can be cooked in the microwave, so it may be worth asking if that is possible. Dhals are good, but not if they have the traditional oil topping – ask if it can be omitted. Go easy on raita as it's likely to have been made with full-fat yoghurt, and most pickles are best refused except for the ones made with plain fresh vegetables like onion or cucumber. Avoid samosas and bhajis, any dishes containing potato or coconut, and all Indian sweets and ice creams.

If you can't resist pizza, choose one with vegetable toppings and share it with friends.

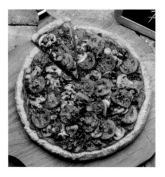

Italian

With the emphasis on pasta and pizza you might think that Italian restaurants would be completely out of the question, but Italian cuisine is actually one of the easiest. There are usually plenty of salads and antipasti that are GI-compatible, and fresh fruit is often available. Go for grilled meat or fish, and antipasti like olives, grilled vegetables or lean cold meats. Never have more than a small slice of thin-based pizza or a small helping of wheat-based, rather than egg, pasta. Always choose vegetable sauces and say no to the Parmesan. Avoid garlic bread unless it's traditional *fettunta* – sourdough with olive oil – and remember not to eat too much if it is. Risottos are out, as are meat cooked in breadcrumbs, polenta, gnocchi, and desserts like tiramisu, panna cotta or rich Italian ice cream.

Japanese
The rice used in sushi does have a lower GI than some other types, but it's still best to keep portions small. Sashimi is raw fish without rice – a much better choice. Avoid vegetable tempura (it's deep-fried), anything coated in breadcrumbs, fried, and anything in rice wrappers.

Mexican
A lot of beans are used in Mexican cookery, so there are usually some possible options. Again, follow the 'plain is best' rule and avoid choosing anything fried, including refried beans. Tortillas are out, as are nachos and rice dishes. Mexican pastries and desserts are way off the GI scale.

Spanish
Tapas can be a good choice for anyone on a GI+GL diet, but watch out for high-fat items. Olives are

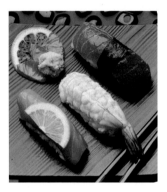

In Japanese restaurants, watch out for the white rice in sushi and the batter on tempura dishes.

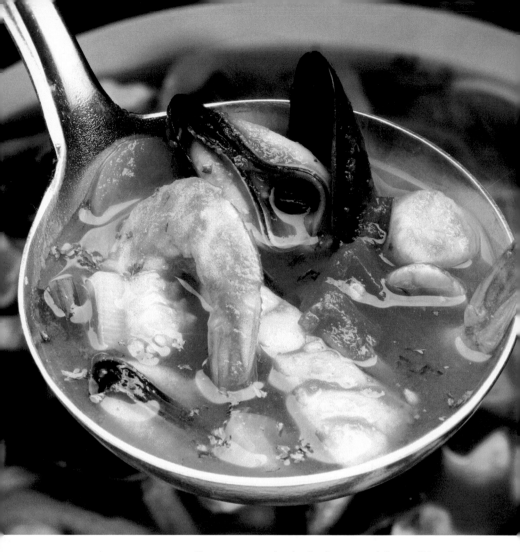

Each region of Spain has its own version of a fish and seafood soup – all of them low GI/GL.

excellent, as are anchovies in vinegar and the traditional Gazpacho soup. Go for grilled meat, fish or seafood and salads. Steer clear of paella and any other dishes based on rice, deep-fried dishes like calamari, anything made with potato, or flan, which is a caramel custard.

Thai

Thai salads are delicious, often containing fish or seafood – go for these. Clear soups with chicken or fish and vegetables, like the classic dish *tom yam pla*, are excellent. Avoid the sticky rice; as with Chinese food, ask for boiled cellophane noodles instead. Soups with rice or noodles get a red light on the GI+GL diet, and it makes sense to avoid any fried foods. Coconut milk, which is popular in Thai cooking, is very high in saturated fat. If you are cooking Thai food at home, always use the low-fat versions available.

Fast food

It is possible to eat in fast food restaurants on a GI+GL diet, but you do need rock-hard self-control. The fat content and calorie levels of most fast food will blow your diet wide open. Stay off anything supersize.

Some menus now have calorie-counted items, but watch out for extras like dressing, which may not be included in the total. That Chicken Caesar Salad could have more calories and fat than a cheeseburger and chips when the creamy dressing is taken into account. Don't add dressings, or any other sauces, and don't help yourself to other people's food (fries can be particularly tempting). If there's a salad bar, avoid mayo-based sauces like thousand island dressing and all salads made with

must know

Think of this
It's easier to resist that quarterpounder with cheese if you remember that you'd have to walk briskly for 10 km, spend over two hours playing tennis or three hours cycling to work off the calories it contains.

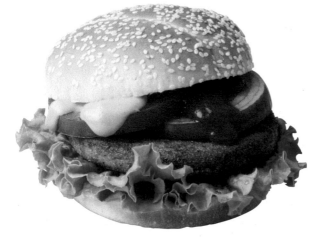

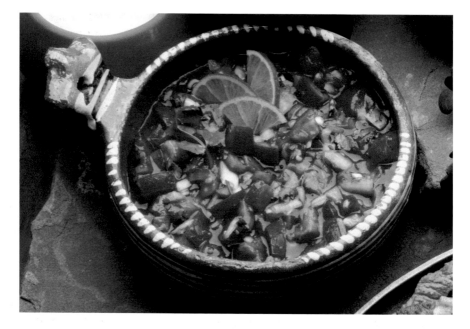

Remember that tomatoes are a powerful superfood that can protect you from cancer.

medium- or high-GI ingredients. Don't even think about ordering chips and automatically remove any batter or breadcrumb coatings on chicken or fish. Don't eat burger buns, either. When it comes to drinks, milkshakes and sweet fizzy drinks are out of sight on the GI/GL scale; your only option may be mineral water.

The traps don't just lie in 'classic' fast food restaurants: a muffin and cappuccino could have a disastrous effect too, totalling about 500 calories. That's about a third of what you would expect to eat in an entire dieting day, all blown on one quickie snack. Even 'skinny' (skimmed milk) cappuccinos and lattes will pack over 100 calories per mug.

One last thing: remember that items which are labelled 'low fat' may be high in sugar. Several fast-food restaurants now serve options labelled 'low-carb', following the popularity of the Atkins diet, but they are frequently high in fats, and therefore in calories too.

Parties

Sticking to your diet at a party can be tricky – apart from anything else, alcohol can affect your judgement and all your good resolutions may vanish. Think about the general guidelines at the beginning of this chapter and eat a good meal before you go, as that will stop you craving food when you get there and, incidentally, slow down the effects of any alcohol on your system.

If dips are available, resist the urge to dip bread or crisps into them – go for raw vegetables – and remember that vegetable salsas and dips based on yoghurt, like tsatsiki, are much lower in calories than fattier dips like taramasalata. Don't eat sausage rolls (the pastry is way, way out) but choose sausages on sticks or chicken drumsticks. And white wine spritzers – wine diluted with fizzy mineral water and lots of ice cubes – are a good choice of drink.

want to know more?

▶ See chapter 9 for the GI/GL ratings of some common foods.
▶ For an American website with good advice on eating out, visit www.low glycemicdiet.com/ smarteating out.htm
▶ You'll also find some handy tips at www.weightloss resources.co.uk/diet /eating_out
▶ There's more advice on dieting and eating out on BUPA's website, although it is not specifically low GI/GL. Go to www.bupa.co.uk and search for 'eating out in a restaurant'.
▶ Check the listings for 'Snacks, nibbles and dips' in *Collins Gem GI* and *GL* guides for the lowdown on lots of potential party problem areas.

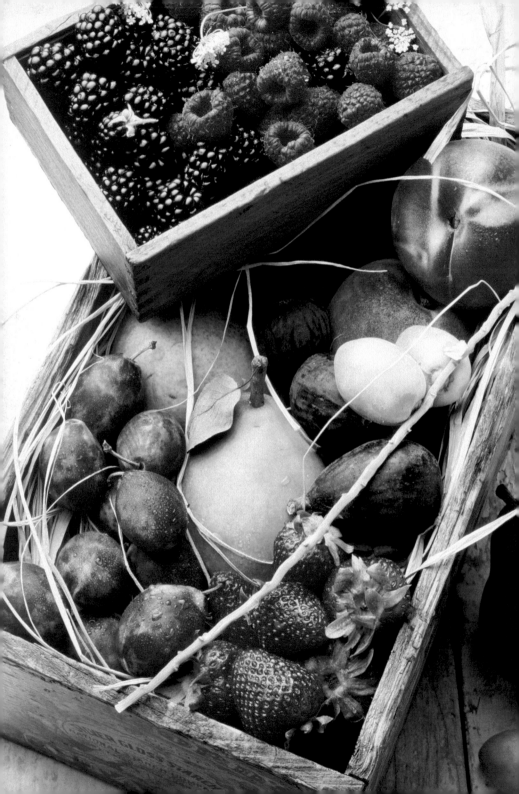

9 Listings

Here's the nitty-gritty. Foods are given a red rating if they are high GI or GL, a yellow rating for medium and a green rating for low. Note that if there is no coloured dot in the GI or GL columns, it's because the food in question doesn't contain carbs, so doesn't have a rating. In addition, the listings supply the carb, calorie, protein and fat count for each food so you can check that you are eating the correct proportion of each type of nutrient. Note: the abbreviation n/a means figures were not available.

Bakery

Most bread, bread products and bakery items are high GI and medium-to-high GL because they are made from refined flour. On a GI+GL diet look out for stoneground, granary or wholemeal bread, but watch out for 'multigrain' which is often made from refined flour. Check the ingredients and compare fibre counts: the higher the fibre, the better. You could also think about making your own; there's a recipe for seeded wholemeal bread on pages 152-3. Shop-bought cakes and biscuits are always going to be bad news– high GI, high GL and full of trans fats.

Nutritional information							
Food type	GI	GL	Carb (g)	Fibre (g)	Cal (kcal)	Pro (g)	Fat (g)
Brown, 1 slice	●	●	12.6	1.7	62	2.5	0.6
Croissant, all butter, each (70g)	●	●	27.8	1.9	261	6.0	14.5
Crumpet, each (50g)	●	●	17.9	–	89	3.6	0.4
Flour, 100g:							
rye, whole	●	●	75.9	n/a	335	8.2	2
wheat, brown	●	●	68.5	n/a	323	12.6	2
wheat, white, breadmaking	●	●	75.3	n/a	341	11.5	1.4
wheat, white, plain	●	●	77.7	n/a	341	9.4	1.3
wheat, white, self-raising	●	●	75.6	n/a	330	8.9	1.2
wheat, wholemeal	●	●	63.9	n/a	310	12.7	2
French stick, 1 slice (2cm thick)	●	●	17.9	1.7	88	3.2	0.9
Granary, 1 slice	●	●	14	1.9	71	2.8	0.8
High-bran, 1 slice	●	●	10.1	2.4	64	3.9	0.8
Naan, plain, half	●	●	29.7	1.7	177	4.7	4.4
Oatcakes, each:							
fine	●	●	6.6	0.9	44	1	1.9

Food type	GI	GL	Carb (g)	Fibre (g)	Cal (kcal)	Pro (g)	Fat (g)
Oatcakes, contd:							
rough	●	●	6.5	0.6	43	1	0.6
Rye crispbread, each:							
dark rye	●	●	5.6	1.7	27	0.9	0.2
multigrain	●	●	6.4	1.8	37	1.3	0.7
original	●	●	5.7	1.6	27	0.8	0.2
sesame	●	●	3.9	1.4	31	0.9	0.6
Pitta bread, medium:							
white	●	●	27.8	1.1	128	4.4	0.6
white with sesame	●	●	24	1.5	131	4.8	1.8
wholewheat	●	●	20.5	3.1	114	5.4	1.2
Pumpernickel, 1 slice	●	●	14.1	1.7	68	2.3	0.5
Rye, 1 slice	●	●	13.7	1.7	66	2.4	0.5
Sourdough, 1 slice	●	●	14.7	0.9	78	2.5	0.9
Stoneground wholemeal,							
1 slice	●	●	11.8	2.2	65	2.9	0.7
Tortillas, each (30g):							
corn	●	●	13.2	–	95	3.0	3.3
flour	●	●	10.3	–	103	3.0	2.0
White, 1 slice	●	●	13.8	1.1	66	2.3	0.6
Wholemeal, 1 slice	●	●	12.9	2.2	66	2.8	0.8

Keep it frozen

Freeze sliced bread and just pull out the slices you need when you need them – it's much easier to resist the temptation to snack on bread that way. The frozen slices can be toasted straight from the freezer.

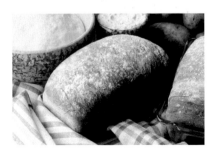

Beans, pulses and cereals

Dried beans have a slightly lower GI than canned beans, and are often cheaper, but they take time to soak and cook. Some will need to be soaked overnight – follow the instructions on the packet. Aduki beans are good for cleansing the system, chick peas contain 'friendly bacteria' to help the digestive system and lentils are a better source of complete proteins than red meat. Most beans are full of B vitamins and fibre, and they're very low in fat. Whatever you use, adding beans to your meal will help slow down your digestion and support your weight-loss diet.

must know

Making baked beans
Avoid the high sugar content of tinned baked beans by combining cooked haricot beans with your own fresh tomato sauce. See also the recipe for chilli beans on page 143.

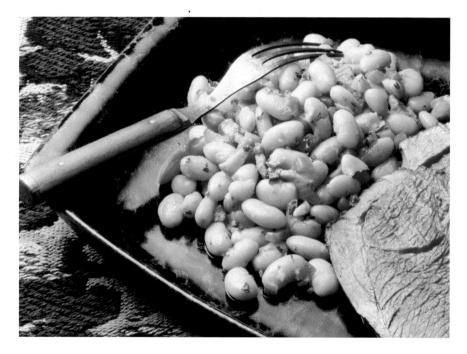

Food type	GI	GL	Carb (g)	Fibre (g)	Cal (kcal)	Pro (g)	Fat (g)
Beans and Pulses							
Aduki beans, 115g	●	●	26	n/a	140	10.6	0.3
Barley, pearl, 100g	●	●	83.6	7.3	360	7.9	1.7
Blackeyed beans, 115g	●	●	23	n/a	133	10	0.8
Bulgur wheat, dry, 100g	●	●	75	1.8	354	11	1.5
Butter beans:							
small can (200g)	●	●	28	10	168	12.8	1
dried, boiled (115g)	●	●	21	5.9	118	8.1	0.7
Chick peas:							
small can (200g)	●	●	32.2	n/a	230	14.4	5.4
dried, boiled (115g)	●	●	20.8	n/a	138	9.6	2.4
Couscous, dry, 100g	●	●	72.5	2	355	23.5	1.9
Haricot beans, 115g							
dried, boiled	●	●	19.6	7	109	7.5	0.6
Lentils, 115g:							
green/brown, boiled	●	●	19.3	n/a	120	10	0.8
red, split, boiled	●	●	20	n/a	114	8.7	0.5
Polenta, ready-made, 100g	●	●	15.7	–	71.9	1.6	0.3
Red kidney beans:							
small can (200g)	●	●	35.6	n/a	200	13.8	1.2
boiled, 115g	●	●	19.8	n/a	118	9.6	0.6
Tofu (soya bean curd), 100g:							
smoked	●	●	1	0.3	148	16	8.9
steamed, fried	●	●	2	–	261	23.5	17.7

Breakfast cereals

Eating breakfast is essential to the success of your diet. Have a good breakfast and it will be much easier to resist sugary mid-morning snacks. Choose cereals containing oats or bran, and without any added sugar or honey coating.

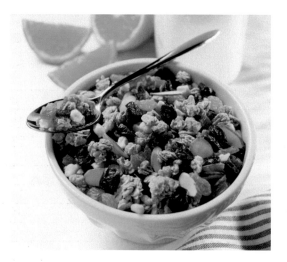

Berry porridge
If you think of porridge without sugar or jam as being rather like wallpaper paste, then try some alternatives. A few dried apricots, chopped and stirred in, or a small spoonful of sultanas are great; even better is a handful of mixed berries. Use them fresh or stir frozen ones in at the end of cooking; the heat will thaw them. If you add them at the beginning you end up with purple porridge...

Food type	GI	GL	Carb (g)	Fibre (g)	Cal (kcal)	Pro (g)	Fat (g)
Bran flakes, 30g	●	○	20.1	4.5	99	3	0.6
Cornflakes, 30g:	●	●	25.3	0.7	111	2.1	0.2
High Fibre Bran, 40g	○	○	18.4	10.8	112	5.6	1.8
Muesli, 50g:			33	3.8	182	5	3.4
apricot	○	○	29.6	2.8	142	3.8	1.8
deluxe	○	○	28.1	5.8	172	5.4	5
high fibre	○	○	35.4	3	158	5.2	3
natural	○	○	31.5	4.3	173	4.8	3.1
organic	○	○	31.2	4.6	190	5	5.1
swiss-style	○	○	36.5	n/a	182	4.9	3
with no added sugar	○	○	33.5	n/a	183	5.2	3.9
Oat Bran Flakes, 30g	○	○	20.1	0.6	99	3	0.6
Oats, 100g:							
instant	○	○	60.4	8.5	359	11	8.1
jumbo	○	○	60.4	8.5	359	11	8.1
rolled	○	○	62	7	368	11	8
Porridge (cooked), 100g:							
made with water	○	○	8.1	0.8	46	1.4	1.1
made with whole milk	○	○	12.6	0.8	113	4.8	5.1
Shredded wheat bisks, 30g:	●	○	19.8	3.4	99	3.4	0.6
bitesize	●	○	20.3	3.5	100	3.4	0.7
sugar coated	●	●	21.6	2.7	105	3	0.6
fruit-filled	●	●	20.7	2.7	96	2.7	0.6
honey nut	●	●	20.6	3	114	3.3	2
Wheat bisks, 30g	○	○	20.3	3.2	102	3.4	0.8

Fruit

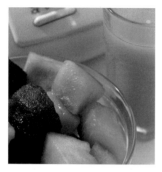

Fructose – fruit sugar – is a natural component of fruit and will affect your blood sugar quite quickly. To minimise the effect of the fructose, eat whole fruits and avoid drinking fruit juices on their own, which would give you an instant blood sugar peak. The GI is lowered if you eat fruit after a main course, or accompanied by a low- or no-GI food. Most fruits remain in the upper end of the low GI/GL category, so don't avoid them – make sure you eat 2 to 3 portions a day for the vitamin C and antioxidants they contain.

Nutritional information

Food type	GI	GL	Carb (g)	Fibre (g)	Cal (kcal)	Pro (g)	Fat (g)
Apple, 1 medium	●	●	21	3.8	82	0.2	0.6
Apricots: 1 fresh	●	●	3.9	0.8	16	0.5	0.1
dried, 8 halves	●	●	9.9	1.7	45	1.1	0.2
Avocado, half medium	●	●	8	3.4	160	1.9	16.4
Banana, 1 medium	●	●	23.2	3.1	95	1.2	0.3
Blackberries:							
fresh, 75g	●	●	3.8	2.3	19	0.7	0.2
Blackcurrants:							
fresh, 75g	●	●	4.9	2.7	21	0.7	–
Blueberries, fresh, 75g	●	●	7.6	1.6	32	0.4	0.2

Nutritional information

Food type	GI	GL	Carb (g)	Fibre (g)	Cal (kcal)	Pro (g)	Fat (g)
Cherries, half cup fresh (90g)	●	●	10.4	0.8	43	0.8	0.09
Clementines, 1 medium	●	●	6.6	0.9	28	0.7	0.1
Dates, quarter cup (50g)	●	●	15.6	0.9	62	0.8	0.05
Figs:							
1 fresh	●	●	9.6	1.7	37	0.4	0.2
dried, ready to eat, 50g	●	●	24.4	0.75	111	1.6	0.75
Grapefruit, half, fresh	●	●	7.8	1.5	34	0.9	0.1
Grapes, black/white, seedless,							
fresh, 75g	●	●	11.6	0.5	45	0.3	0.75
Guavas, fresh, 60g	●	●	3	2.2	16	0.5	0.3
Kiwi fruit, peeled, each	●	●	10.6	1.9	49	1.1	0.5
Lemon, whole	●	●	3.2	N	19	1	0.3
Mangos, 1 medium	●	●	16	0.2	66	0.8	0.2
Melon, fresh, medium slice:							
cantaloupe	●	●	4.8	1.3	22	0.7	0.1
galia	●	●	6.4	0.5	27	0.6	0.1
honeydew	●	●	7.5	0.7	32	0.7	0.1
watermelon	●	●	8.1	0.1	35	0.6	0.3
Nectarines, 1 medium	●	●	13.5	1.8	60	2.1	0.1
Oranges, 1 medium	●	●	12.8	2.5	56	1.6	0.1
Papaya, half, fresh	●	●	10	2.5	41	0.6	0.1
Peach, 1 medium	●	●	11.4	2.2	50	1.3	0.1
Pear, 1 medium	●	●	15	3.3	60	0.4	0.1
Pineapple, fresh, 60g	●	●	6.0	0.3	25	0.2	0.1
Plums, 1 medium	●	●	8.8	1.6	36	0.6	0.1
Raspberries, fresh, 60g	●	●	2.8	1.5	15	0.8	0.2
Satsumas, 1 medium	●	●	12.8	2	54	1.4	0.1
Strawberries, 70g	●	●	4.2	0.8	19	0.6	0.07
Tangerines, fresh, one	●	●	8	1.3	35	0.9	0.1

Meat and poultry

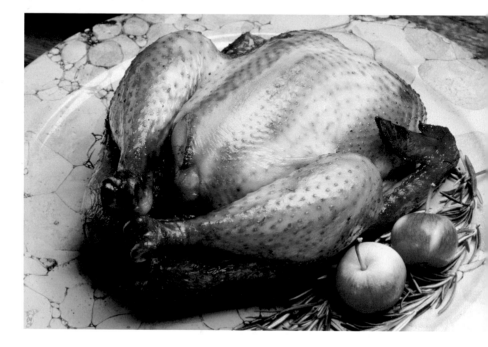

Fresh and frozen meat and poultry don't contain carbs and so have no GI unless they've been processed – made into something like sausage, burger or luncheon meat, or coated in breadcrumbs. Avoid these if possible. Remove any visible fat before cooking, or it could melt into the meat. Whatever meat you are eating, watch out for calorie levels and saturated fat content and remember the portion control rules – no more than a quarter of your plate should be covered by meat or poultry.

must know

Snip the skin

Chicken skin contains a lot of saturated fat, so remove it before cooking. Snip the edge of the skin with scissors, then pull it away from the meat.

Nutritional information

Food type	GI	GL	Carb (g)	Fibre (g)	Cal (kcal)	Pro (g)	Fat (g)
Bacon, 3 rashers, back (50g):							
dry fried			–	–	148	12.1	11
grilled			–	–	144	11.6	10.8
Beef, 100g:							
rump steak, lean, grilled			–	–	177	31	5.9
rump steak, lean, fried			–	–	183	30.9	6.6
topside, lean & fat, roasted			–	–	244	32.8	12.5
sausages, 2, grilled	●	●	14.7	n/a	313	15	21.9
beefburgers, 100g, fried			0.1	–	326	28.5	23.9
Chicken, 100g:							
breast, grilled			–	–	148	32	2.2
breast, stir fried			–	–	161	29.7	4.6
light & dark meat, roasted			–	–	177	27.3	7.5
light meat, roasted			–	–	153	30.2	3.6
cold roast chicken, breast meat, 50g			–	–	76	15.1	1.8
Ham, 50g:							
honey-roast	●	●	1.4	0.5	68	10	2.2
on the bone	●	●	0.4	0.3	68	10.4	7.7
Parma	●	●	0.05	0	120	12.5	7.5
Lamb, 100g:							
loin chops, lean & fat, grilled			–	–	305	26.5	22.1
leg, lean & fat, roasted			–	–	240	28.1	14.2
Pork, 100g:							
loin chops, lean, grilled			–	–	184	31.6	6.4
leg, lean only, roasted			–	–	182	33	5.5
sausages, 2, grilled			11	n/a	347	15.5	26.9
Turkey, 100g:	●	●					
breast fillet, grilled			–	–	155	35	1.7
dark meat, roasted			–	–	177	29.4	6.6

Nuts, seeds and dried fruit

Nuts are often recommended as a suitable GI- and GL-friendly snack, but they are very high in calories, so you have to be careful about how many you eat – a 25g portion could be as few as 6 nuts. Pistachios in their shells are an excellent choice – partly because taking them out of the shells will slow you down! Black or green olives, or some dried fruits, are a lower-calorie, nutritionally healthy alternative snack.

must know

Nuts on top

Toast chopped nuts in a dry frying pan, stirring them until they darken, and then sprinkle them on top of soup, no-fat Greek yoghurt or salads. Walnuts are particularly good served with baby spinach leaves.

Nutritional information

Food type	GI	GL	Carb (g)	Fibre (g)	Cal (kcal)	Pro (g)	Fat (g)
Almonds:							
weighed with shells, 50g	●	●	1.3	1.4	115	5.2	5.2
Apple rings, 25g	●	●	15	2.4	60	0.5	0.1
Apricots, 25g	●	●	9.1	n/a	39.5	1	0.15
Banana chips, 25g	●	●	15	0.3	128	0.3	7.9
Brazils:							
weighed with shells, 50g	●	●	0.7	1.9	157	3.3	15.7
Cashews:							
kernel only, 25g	●	●	4.5	0.8	144	4.5	12
Currants, 25g	●	●	17	n/a	67	0.6	0.1
Dates, flesh & skin, 25g	●	●	17	n/a	68	0.8	0.1
Figs, 25g	●	●	13.2	n/a	57	0.9	0.4
Hazelnuts:							
weighed with shell, 50g	●	●	1.2	1.3	124	1.4	6

Food type	GI	GL	Carb (g)	Fibre (g)	Cal (kcal)	Pro (g)	Fat (g)
Hazelnuts, contd:							
kernel only, 25g	●	●	1.5	1.5	167	4.3	16
Macadamia nuts, salted, 50g	●	●	2.7	n/a	374	4	2.7
Olives, 15g black			3.4	1.7	32	0.2	1.0
Peanuts:							
plain, kernel only, 25g	●	●	3.1	n/a	141	6.5	11.5
dry roasted, 50g	●	●	5.2	n/a	295	12.9	24.8
roasted & salted, 50g	●	●	3.6	n/a	301	12.4	26.5
Pine nuts, kernel only, 25g	●	●	1	n/a	172	3.5	17.2
Pineapple, diced, 25g	●	●	8.4	2	69	0.6	0.3
Pistachios, weighed with							
shells, 50g	●	●	2.3	1.7	83	2.5	7.7
Pumpkin seeds, 25g	●	●	11.8	1.1	143	7.3	12
Raisins, seedless, 25g	●	●	17.3	n/a	68	0.5	0.1
Sultanas, 25g	●	●	7.3	n/a	69	0.7	0.1
Sunflower seeds, 25g	●	●	4.7	3	149	5.9	11.9
Walnuts:							
weighed with shell, 50g	●	●	0.7	0.8	148	3.2	14.7
halves , 25g	●	●	0.8	0.9	172	3.7	17.1

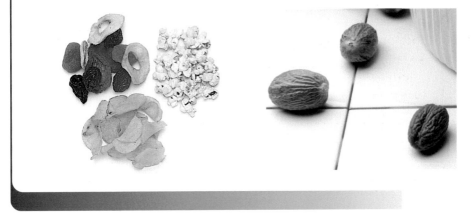

Pasta

Most pasta is either at the top end of low GI, or has a medium medium GI but high GL: even an average portion will have an impact on your blood sugar levels. Wholemeal pasta is preferable, with a GI of just 37, and it isn't as stodgy as it used to be. Keep portion sizes small – not more than 40g dry weight per person, which will make around 100g when cooked. Avoid bottled pasta sauces as the sugar and oil content are often high. It's easy to make your own basic tomato sauce with garlic, chopped tomatoes and fresh basil.

must know

With a bite
Keep pasta 'al dente' – with a bit of a bite to it. Not only is that how it's supposed to be, but the digestive system also has to do more work to break it down.

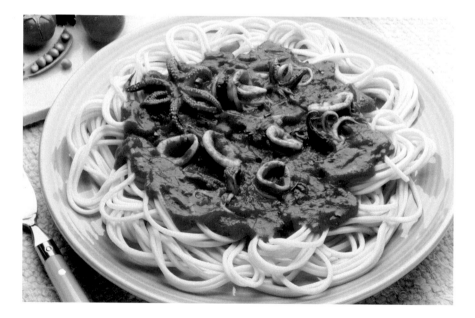

Food type	GI	GL	Carb (g)	Fibre (g)	Cal (kcal)	Pro (g)	Fat (g)
Dried pasta shapes,							
cooked weight 100g:							
standard	●	●	18.1	–	89	3.1	0.4
verdi	●	●	18.3	–	93	3.2	0.4
Fresh egg pasta, 100g:							
spaghetti	●	●	24	1	129	5	1.4
tagliatelle	●	●	24	1	129	5	1
Lasagne sheets, cooked weight 100g	●	●	18.1	–	89	3.1	0.4
Spaghetti, cooked weight 100g:							
dried, egg	●	●	22.2	n/a	104	3.6	0.7
wholemeal	●	●	23.2	n/a	113	4.7	0.9

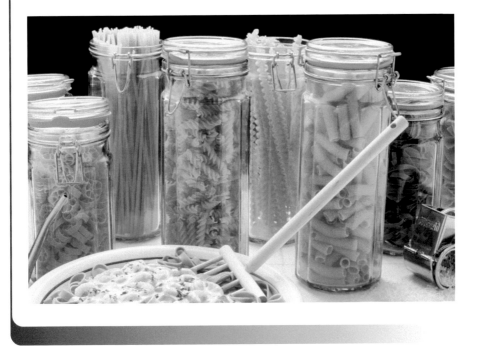

Rice and noodles

Be careful with rice, as it is either high or medium GI and high GL. Don't use ready noodles, easy-cook rice or the sticky rice so popular in Thai cooking. Go for basmati, brown or long-grain rice or mung bean noodles (GI 39). Remember portions of rice or noodles should only cover a quarter of your plate.

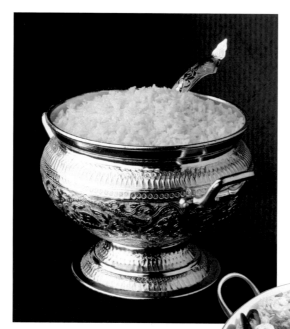

Nutritional information

Food type	GI	GL	Carb (g)	Fibre (g)	Cal (kcal)	Pro (g)	Fat (g)
Arborio rice, 75g	●	●	23.3	0.3	105	2.2	0.3
Basmati rice, 75g	○	●	22.7	–	103	2.7	0.2
Brown rice, 75g	○	●	24	0.6	106	2	0.6
Egg fried rice, 75g	○	●	19.2	0.3	156	2	8
Egg noodles, 75g	○	○	9.8	0.5	47	2	0.4
Long grain rice, 75g	○	●	22.6	–	103	2.1	0.3
Pilau rice, 75g	●	●	23	0.5	106	2.7	0.4
Short grain rice, 75g	●	●	26	0.7	108	2	0.3
Thai rice noodles, 75g	●	●	26	0.7	108	2	0.3
Thread noodles, 75g	○	○	7.4	–	51	1.8	1.5
White rice, plain, 75g	●	●	3.2	0.1	104	2	0.1
Wholegrain rice, 75g	○	●	21.2	0.6	102	2.7	0.7

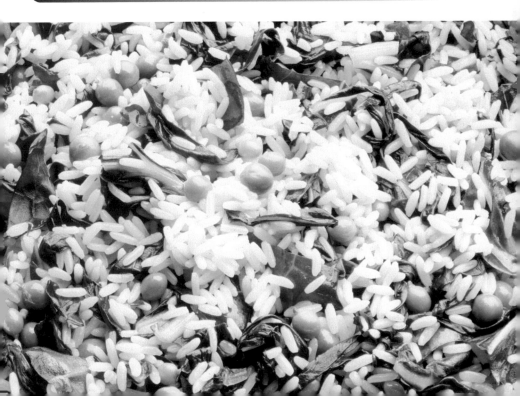

Vegetables

Almost all fresh vegetables are good news for GI+GL dieters. Potatoes are the main problem area; stick to new ones, cooked in their skins, and avoid others – or choose sweet potatoes as an alternative. One or two vegetables have very different GI and GL ratings – pumpkin and turnips, for example – because of the portion sizes used in GI testing.

must know

Sweet potatoes
Sweet potatoes aren't just great because of their relatively low GI; they're packed with useful antioxidants too. Use them in any family favourite dishes where you would normally use potatoes: shepherd's pie, cottage pie, fish pie, or moussaka.

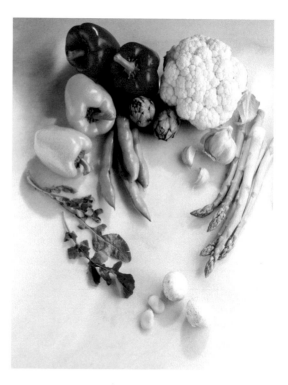

Nutritional information

Food type	GI	GL	Carb (g)	Fibre (g)	Cal (kcal)	Pro (g)	Fat (g)
Artichokes, 1 globe	●	●	2.7	–	18	2.8	0.2
Asparagus, 6 spears, boiled	●	●	3.8	1.5	21	2.4	0.3
Aubergine, half medium, fried	●	●	1.4	n/a	151	0.6	16
Avocado, half	●	●	8	n/a	160	1.9	14
Beans, broad, boiled, 75g	●	●	4.2	4.0	36	3.8	0.6
Beans, French, 100g boiled	●	●	2.9	n/a	22	1.8	0.5
Beans, runner, 50g, trimmed,							
boiled	●	●	1.1	n/a	9	0.6	0.2
Beetroot, 90g:							
pickled	●	●	5.0	n/a	25	1.1	0.2
boiled	●	●	8.6	n/a	41	2.0	0.1
Broccoli, florets, boiled, 60g	●	●	0.6	n/a	14	1.9	0.5
Brussels sprouts, 6 trimmed,							
boiled	●	●	10.9	n/a	49	3.3	0.6
Cabbage (Savoy, Summer), 75g:							
trimmed	●	●	3.1	n/a	20	1.3	0.3
shredded & boiled	●	●	1.7	n/a	12	0.75	0.3
Spring greens, raw	●	●	2.3	n/a	25	2.3	0.7
Spring greens, boiled	●	●	1.2	n/a	15	1.4	0.5
white	●	●	3.7	n/a	20	1.0	0.2
Carrot:							
1 medium, raw	●	●	7.9	n/a	35	0.6	0.3
1 medium, raw (young)	●	●	6.9	n/a	34	0.8	2.7
grated, 40g	●	●	3.2	1	15	0.2	0.1
boiled (frozen), 80g	●	●	3.8	1.8	18	0.3	0.2
boiled (young), 80g	●	●	3.5	n/a	18	0.5	0.3
Cassava, 100g:							
baked	●	●	40.1	1.7	155	0.7	0.2
boiled	●	●	33.5	1.4	130	0.5	0.2

Food type	GI	GL	Carb (g)	Fibre (g)	Cal (kcal)	Pro (g)	Fat (g)
Cauliflower, 100g:							
raw	●	●	3.0	n/a	34	3.6	0.9
boiled	●	●	2.1	n/a	28	2.9	0.9
Celeriac, 100g:							
flesh only, boiled	●	●	1.9	3.2	15	0.9	0.5
Celery, 100g:							
stem only, raw	●	●	0.9	n/a	7	0.5	0.2
stem only, boiled	●	●	0.8	n/a	8	0.5	0.3
Corn-on-the-cob							
boiled, 1 medium cob	●	●	22.4	n/a	127	4.8	2.6
Courgettes (zucchini):							
trimmed, raw 50g	●	●	0.9	n/a	9	0.9	0.2
trimmed, boiled, 75g	●	●	1.5	n/a	14	1.5	0.3
Cucumber, trimmed, 75g	●	●	1.1	n/a	7.5	0.5	0.1
Fennel, Florence, *boiled,* 75g	●	●	1.1	n/a	8	0.7	0.1
Garlic, half tsp purée or							
1 clove, crushed	●	●	1.9	0.9	60	0.1	5.7
Ginger root, half tsp, grated	●	●	1	n/a	5	0.2	–
Kale, curly, boiled, 40g	●	●	0.4	n/a	10	0.9	0.4
Leeks, *boiled,* 100g	●	●	2.6	n/a	21	1.2	0.7
Lettuce, 1 cup (30g):							
green	●	●	0.5	0.3	4	0.2	0.1
iceberg	●	●	0.6	n/a	4	0.2	0.1
mixed leaf	●	●	0.9	0.8	5.1	0.3	0.03
Mediterranean salad leaves	●	●	0.9	0.5	5.7	0.3	0.1
spinach, rocket & watercress	●	●	0.4	0.4	7.5	0.9	0.3
Mange-tout, 50g:							
raw	●	●	2.1	n/a	16	1.8	0.1
boiled	●	●	1.6	n/a	13	1.6	0.05

Food type	GI	GL	Carb (g)	Fibre (g)	Cal (kcal)	Pro (g)	Fat (g)
Mushrooms, common, 40g:							
raw	●	●	0.2	n/a	5	0.7	0.2
boiled	●	●	0.2	0.4	4	0.7	0.1
Mushrooms, oyster, 30g	●	●	0	0.06	2.4	0.5	0.06
Okra (gumbo, ladies' fingers):							
raw, 25g	●	●	0.8	n/a	8	0.7	0.2
boiled, 30g	●	●	0.8	n/a	8	0.7	0.2
Onions:	●	●					
raw, flesh only, 30g	●	●	2.4	n/a	11	0.4	0.1
boiled, 40g	●	●	1.5	0.3	7	0.2	–
Parsnips, trimmed, peeled,	●	●					
boiled, 80g	●	●	10.3	n/a	53	1.3	1.0
Peas:	●	●					
fresh, raw, 75g	●	●	8.5	n/a	62	5.1	1.1
boiled, 90g	●	●	9.0	n/a	71	6.0	1.4
Peppers:	●	●					
green, raw, 40g	●	●	1.0	n/a	6	0.3	0.1
green, boiled, 50g	●	●	1.3	n/a	9	0.5	0.2
red, raw, 40g	●	●	2.6	n/a	13	0.4	0.2
red, boiled, 50g	●	●	3.5	n/a	17	0.6	0.2
yellow, raw, 40g	●	●	2.1	0.7	10	0.5	0.1
chilli, 15g	●	●	0.1	n/a	3	0.4	0.1
Potatoes, new, 100g:							
boiled, peeled	●	●	17.8	n/a	75	1.5	0.3
boiled in skins	●	●	15.4	n/a	66	1.4	0.3
Potatoes, old, 90g:							
baked, flesh & skin	●	●	28.5	n/a	122	3.5	0.2
baked, flesh only	●	●	16.2	n/a	69	2.0	0.1
boiled, peeled	●	●	15.3	n/a	65	1.6	0.1

Food type	GI	GL	Carb (g)	Fibre (g)	Cal (kcal)	Pro (g)	Fat (g)
Pumpkin, flesh only, boiled, 75g	●	●	1.6	n/a	10	0.4	0.2
Raddicchio, 30g	●	●	0.5	–	4	0.4	0.1
Radish, red, 6	●	●	1.1	n/a	7	0.4	0.1
Radish, white/mooli, 20g	●	●	0.6	n/a	3	0.2	0.02
Shallots, 30g	●	●	1.0	n/a	6	0.4	0.2
Spinach:							
raw, one cup, 30g	●	●	0.5	n/a	7	0.8	0.2
boiled, 90g	●	●	0.7	n/a	17	2.0	0.7
frozen, boiled, 90g	●	●	0.4	n/a	19	2.8	0.7
Spring onions, bulbs & tops, 30g	●	●	0.9	n/a	7	0.6	0.2
Squash:							
flesh only, 50g	●	●	1.1	n/a	6	0.2	0.1
flesh only, boiled, 75g	●	●	1.2	n/a	7	0.3	0.1
Swede, flesh only, boiled, 90g	●	●	2.0	n/a	10	0.3	0.1
Sweet potato, boiled, 90g	●	●	18.4	n/a	76	1.0	0.3

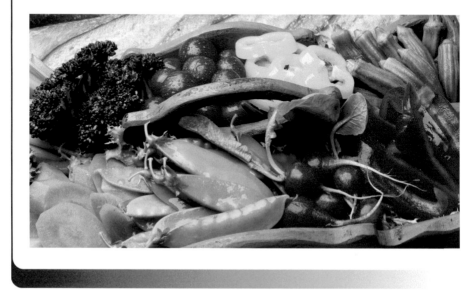

Food type	GI	GL	Carb (g)	Fibre (g)	Cal (kcal)	Pro (g)	Fat (g)
Sweetcorn, kernels, 80g	●	●	21.3	n/a	97	2.3	1.0
Tomatoes:							
1 medium	●	●	0.5	0.07	3.2	0.13	0.07
canned, whole, 100g	●	●	3	n/a	16	1	0.1
cherry, 6	●	●	5.2	1.6	31	1.2	0.8
Turnip, flesh only, boiled, 60g	●	●	2.8	n/a	7	0.4	0.2
Water chestnuts, canned, 40g	●	●	1.9	1	11.2	0.7	0.1
Yam, flesh only, boiled, 90g	●	●	29.7	n/a	120	1.5	0.3

must know

Buy organic

Organic vegetables may be more expensive, but remember that you are avoiding pesticide residues. Numerous studies now indicate that chemical fertilisers are absorbed by our bodies and don't do us any good. Organic produce usually tastes better as an added bonus!

Further reading

General nutrition

Bodyfoods for Busy People,
Jane Clarke, 2004

Collins Gem Calorie Counter,
2004

Collins Gem Carb Counter,
2004

Collins Gem GI, 2005

Collins Gem Healthy Eating,
1999

Collins Gem What Diet?, 2005

Eat Well, Live Well series,
recipe books, various
authors

Fat is a Feminist Issue, Susie
Orbach, 1998

Food Pharmacy, Jean Carper,
2000

A Good Life, Leo Hickman,
2005

Greek Doctor's Diet, Fedon
Alexander Lindberg, 2005

Healthy Eating for Diabetics,
Antony Worrall Thompson
& Azmina Govindji, 2003

Jane Clarke's Bodyfoods
Cookbook: Recipes for Life,
Jane Clarke, 2001

L is for Label: How to Read
Between the Lines on Food
Packaging, Amanda Ursell,
2004

Nutrition for Life, Ian W.
Campbell, 2005

Patrick Holford's New
Optimum Nutrition Bible,
Patrick Holford, 2004

Think Well to be Well, Azmina
Govindji, 2002

The Vegetarian Low-Carb Diet,
Rose Elliott, 2005

Vitamins and Minerals
Handbook, Amanda Ursell
et al, 2001

You Are What You Eat
Cookbook, Dr Gillian
McKeith, 2005

The GI/GL diet

The GI Diet, by Rick Gallop,
2004

The GI Diet – Shopping and
Eating Out Pocket Guide, by
Rick Gallop, 2005

Living the GI Diet: To Maintain
Healthy, Permanent Weight
Loss, Rick Gallop, 2004

The GI Guide, Rick Gallop and
Hamish Renton, 2005

The Low GI Diet, by Jennie
Brand-Miller & Kaye
Foster-Powell with
Joanna McMillan-Price,
2004

The Complete Guide to GI
Values, Jennie Brand-Miller,
Kaye Foster-Powell & Dr
Susanna Holt, 2004

The Low GI Life Plan, by
Jennie Brand-Miller & Kaye
Foster-Powell, 2004

The Low GI Diet, Jennie
Brand-Miller, 2005

Easy GI Diet, by Helen Foster,
2004

The High-Energy Cookbook, by
Rachael Anne Hill, 2004

The GI Plan, by Azmina
Govindji & Nina Puddefoot,
2004

The G-Index Diet, by Richard
Podell & William Proctor,
1994

Antony Worrall Thompson's GI
Diet, by Antony Worrall
Thompson, 2005

The Fat Busting GI Angel,
Gunter Schaule, 2003

The Simple 0-10 GI Diet,
Azmina Govindji and Nina
Puddefoot, 2005

The Healthy Low GI and Low
Carb Diet, Charles Clark,
Maureen Clark, 2005

The Holford Diet, Patrick
Holford, 2005

The Holford Diet Low-GL
Cookbook, Patrick Holford &
Fiona Macdonald Joyce,
2005

The GL Diet, Nigel Denby,
2005

Need to know more?

British Dietetic Association
5th Floor, Charles House
148/9 Great Charles Street
Birmingham B3 3HT
0121 200 8080
www.bda.uk.com

British Heart Foundation
14 Fitzhardinge Street
London W1H 6DH
0845 070 8070
www.bhf.org.uk

British Nutrition Foundation
High Holborn House
52-54 High Holborn
London WC1V 6RQ
020 7404 6504
www.nutrition.org.uk

Coronary Prevention Group
2 Taviton Street
London WC1H 0BT
020 7927 2125
www.healthnet.org

Diabetes UK
10 Parkway
London NW1 7AA
Careline 0845 1202960
or 020 7424 1000
www.diabetes.co.uk

Weight Concern
Brook House
2-6 Torrington Place
London WC1E 7HN
020 7679 6636
www.weightconcern.com

Picture credits

Appendices

Index